Competitive Cycling

Achim Schmidt

Competitive Cycling

Meyer & Meyer Sport

British Library Cataloguing in Publication Data

A catalogue record for this book is available from the British Library

Competitive Cycling

Maidenhead: Meyer & Meyer Sport (UK) Ltd., 1998

2nd revised edition 2014 of *Handbook of Competitive Cycling*

ISBN: 978-1-78255-033-4

© 1998 by Meyer & Meyer Sport (UK) Ltd.

2nd revised edition 2014 of *Handbook of Competitive Cycling*

Aachen, Auckland, Beirut, Budapest, Cairo, Cape Town, Dubai, Hägendorf,

Indianapolis, Singapore, Sydney, Tehran, Wien

Member of the World Sport Publishers' Association (WSPA)

Printed by: B.O.S.S Druck und Medien GmbH

ISBN: 978-1-78255-033-4

E-Mail: info@m-m-sports.com

www.m-m-sports.de

Contents

Foreword

Cycling is experiencing a boom. There are more and more racing cyclists, the cyclosportive scene is growing, and licensed races are more and more popular. Many women have discovered that cycling is the ideal sport that allows them to leave everyday life behind and ride to their heart's content come rain or shine. Cycling is definitely one of the most attractive sports and can be pursued well into old age.

This book aims to bring the excitement and variety of road cycling closer to the reader and to answer many questions on cycling from amateur to professional cycle racing. Anyone who is interested in more specific training questions will notice that this clearly structured topic is very complex and that performances on the bike can be planned but are not predictable. No training plan can guarantee success, for many different training methods can lead to a race victory, even a World Championship title. Anyone who takes cycling seriously and trains conscientiously is definitely on the road to success and won't have to resort to medical assistance. Unfortunately, too many cycling pros and even amateurs take the easy way and resort to some drugs, without really knowing if they might permanently damage their health.

I hope you really enjoy your cycling and that this book helps you plan your personal training program without needing to resort to doping.

Königsdorf, Achim Schmidt

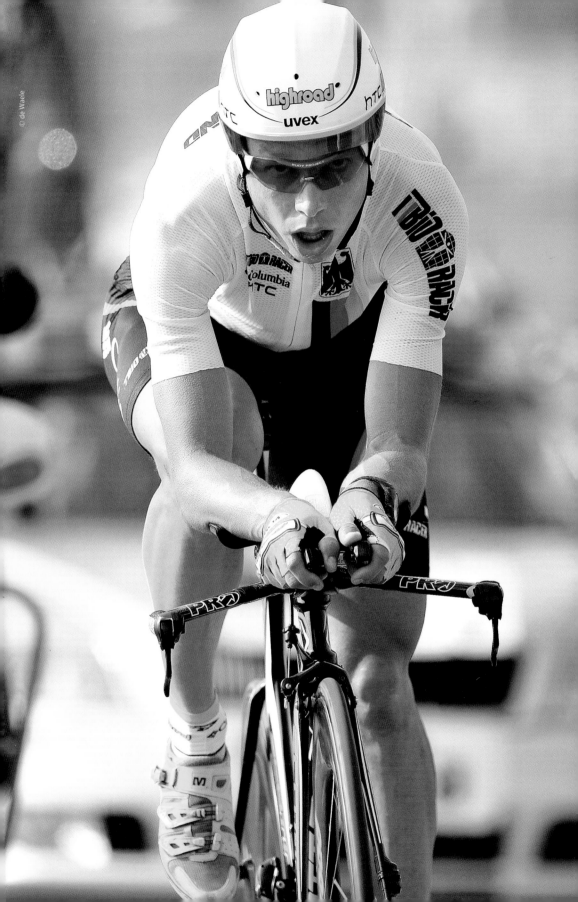

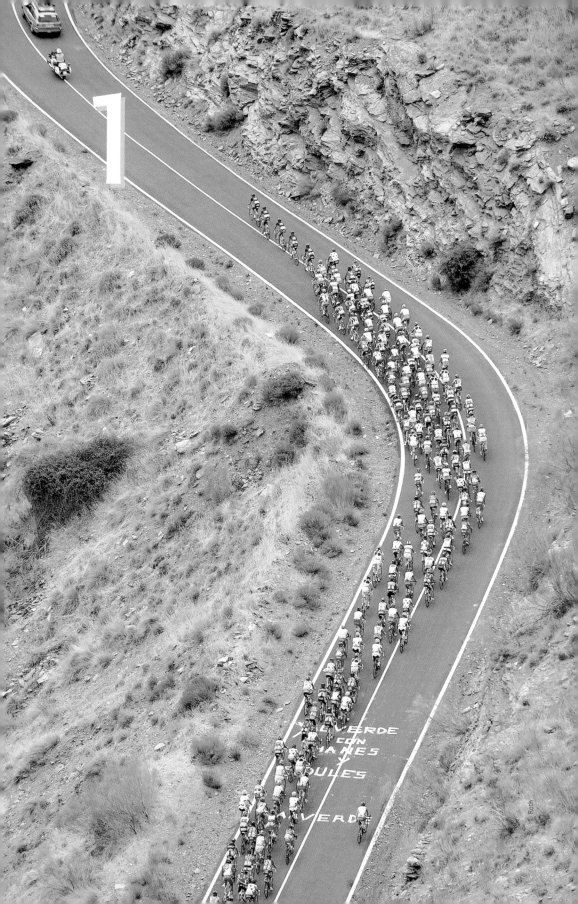

1

1   Introduction

1.1   About the Book

This book on road cycling addresses important subject areas for cyclists, recreational and especially competitive cyclists. The information is well-founded and presented in an easy-to-understand way, without going into scientific detail.

Each chapter is organized and structured so that it progresses from one topic to the next, including the medical and training science sections. Readers without the relevant previous knowledge will therefore find it hard to understand one chapter read in isolation. So take the time to read through those chapters and sections that present the theoretical principles of cycling carefully, as this is a prerequisite for understanding the complex training processes.

What may at first seem very complicated is in most cases explained in very simple terms. Readers are given sufficient information and knowledge to help them make informed judgments on their training and the training of others; they should use a combination of their own experiences and the information in the book to arrive at their own individual training style. Unfortunately, it has only been possible to outline a few topics briefly in this book, but these topics are addressed more comprehensively elsewhere for those who are interested.

What is the secret? The fact is there is no secret recipe for success, no magic training plan, no new secret way of reaching peak form. Top road cycling performances are a product of countless individual factors, many of which are covered in this book, and the most important of which are many years of intensive training and talent.

For example, many cyclists seem to think that peak performance is guaranteed by sticking to a certain training heart rate. However, knowing and understanding the different zones, how to determine them accurately and how to combine these zones and training methods within a periodized training plan, will lead to success. The same is true for purported "miracle foods," as well as the often overrated influence of equipment on overall performance.

Listen to your body: More important than all scientific and theoretical information is what your body tells you. This is usually the best indicator of performance levels and training planning. Modern sport is now more and more technical and even commercialized, and both increasingly distance it from its original purpose of providing enjoyment, variety, health, and a quality of life. Sports ethics have long been an issue in the doping-ridden sport of cycling.

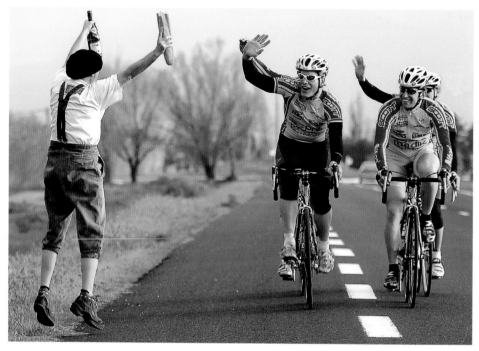

Training is fun!

It really isn't necessary to pump your body full of performance-enhancing substances to achieve great performances and to be successful.

The time has come to take stock and see the sport for what it is to enable high-performance cycling to emerge from its current impasse and to continue to develop.

1.2   Cycling as a Popular Health Pursuit

Over the last few years, cycling has undergone an unprecedented boom. While cycling as a means of transport has increased dramatically and many cities are recording an increase in bicycle traffic, the actual sport of cycling has grown more and more popular. Never before have so many people turned to cycling, whether on a racing bike, trekking bike, fitness, or mountain bike, as a leisure activity.

Many new cycling enthusiasts have become interested in cycling as a sport via mountain biking. Many mountain bikers now also ride road-racing bikes, and cyclosportive or gran fondo races are increasingly popular and widespread. Cycling as a mass sport has a number of advantages, all of which lead to an improved quality of life. In particular when it comes to the growing problem of first world diseases (e.g., arteriosclerosis, obesity), cycling improves health, not only because of the exercise itself, but also because it encourages a healthier lifestyle in general. Practicing a sport often leads to a change in consciousness that in turn leads to a healthier lifestyle, thus stopping, or at least reducing to an acceptable level, the destructive effect a sedentary lifestyle, poor diet, nicotine, and alcohol has on the body. This coupled with the enjoyment of cycling through the countryside leads to a significantly improved feeling of well-being.

For many recreational athletes, cycling in the countryside is not just an individual sport but also a social activity that enables them to meet new people or maintain existing friendships via therapeutic groups, ride-outs, and clubs.

For all these reasons, cycling for many people represents the opportunity to switch off and be alone, away from the stresses of everyday life, leaving their cares and worries behind. If it is hard to find time for yourself in your family or professional life, it is always possible at any time on your bike.

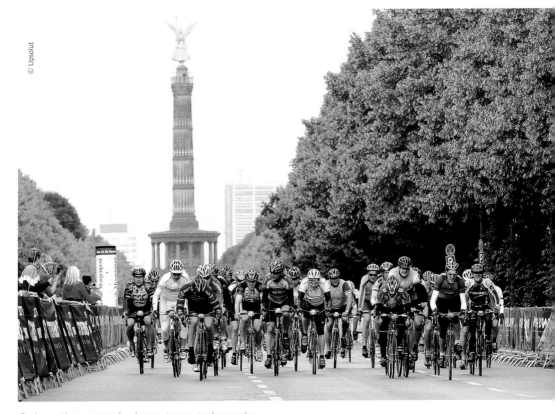

© Upsolut

Cyclosportives or gran fondos are increasingly popular.

So cycling not only positively affects your body and health, but it also increases mental well-being by allowing you to distance yourself from your everyday problems.

Cycling holidays are also an increasingly popular pursuit. While in a car we experience the countryside as observers through a window, on a bike we are able to experience it directly.

1.3   Cycling as a Performance Sport

Most of the above-mentioned advantages of cycling at a recreational level also apply at competitive and high-performance levels. While performance and competition are usually low on the agenda for recreational cyclists, they take on a much greater importance for competitive cyclists.

Racing cyclists must cope with extremely hard training and pain in training and racing. Apart from a few extreme sports (e.g., multiple ultratriathlons, 100-km races), cycle racing is the most demanding sport in terms of endurance performance, not just on a single day. The Tour de France, for example, lasts for three exhausting weeks, which pushes the cyclists' bodies to their limits. Cycle racing reveals the amazing adaptability of the human body to endurance training (see chapter 2). However, cycling as a performance sport is experiencing a crisis thanks to the doping problems that insiders have long been aware of. But like a relapsed alcoholic, the sport of cycling carries on drinking regardless, sinking deeper and deeper into a depression that is not limited to the pro circuit. Cycling clubs are finding it harder and harder to find youngsters who are prepared to practice their sport, with or without questionable role models.

As a result, entries for youth races are dwindling. Sponsors are turning to other sports, and cycle races are being cancelled. Nobody knows how cycling can break away from this vicious cycle, but top riders are continuing to dope, which is pushing an entire sport nearer to the edge of the abyss.

However, luckily some clubs are proving that children and adolescents can still be inspired to take up cycling. With innovative concepts, these clubs manage to get many youngsters in their regions involved in cycling. This new spirit of cycling must spread more widely to give the sport a more positive outlook for the future.

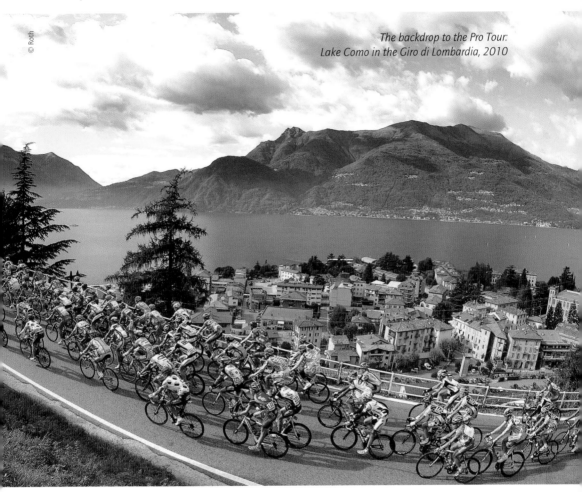

The backdrop to the Pro Tour:
Lake Como in the Giro di Lombardia, 2010

© Roth

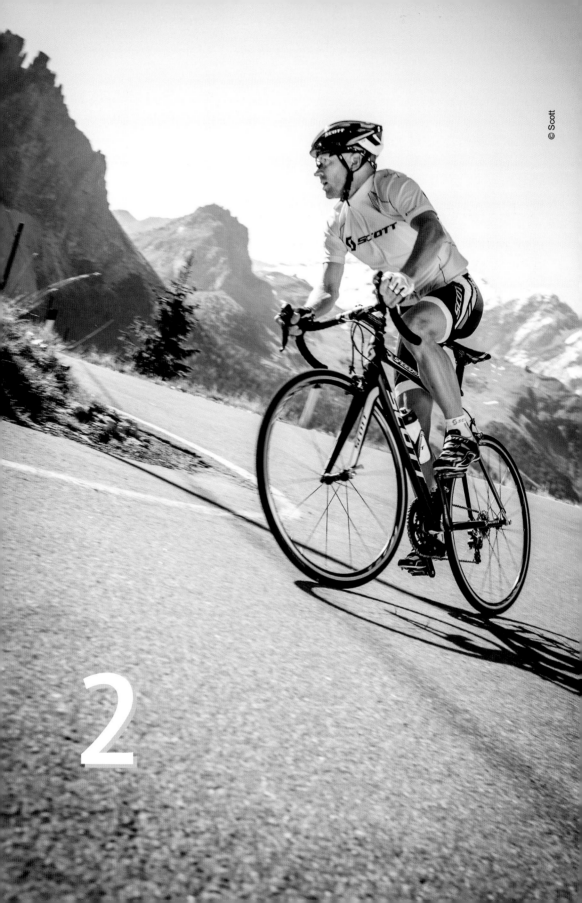

2

2 Anatomical and Physiological Principles of Cycling

2.1 Anatomical and Physiological Principles

The aim of this chapter is to explain the structure and function of the human body when cycling. Processes from muscle contraction to digestion are described in simple form in order to develop an understanding of how our bodies work, as this is essential in order to gain a good understanding of the training process and to be able to understand and evaluate the pros and cons of certain training content.

Musculoskeletal system

Our journey through the body should start with the muscles, bones and joints, in other words, the musculoskeletal system. We only realize the importance of a smoothly functioning musculoskeletal system when movements become painful or even impossible due to sprains, bruises, or at worst even tears or fractures. Even simple muscle soreness can significantly reduce an athlete's ability to train.

Muscles

The over 600 muscles in the human body normally make up 40% of bodyweight in men and around 25% in women and at rest consume about 20% of the resting metabolic rate. At maximal effort (peak athletic performance), this figure soars to up to 90%.

Muscles have the ability to convert chemical energy (food) into mechanical energy (contraction), just like a combustion engine. A muscle or muscle group never works in isolation but is always dependent on one or more opposing muscles (antagonists).

For example: In the leg, the hamstrings (agonists) are situated opposite the quadriceps (antagonists). There are two fundamentally different types of muscle action:

    a. Static
    b. Dynamic

Static means without movement. On the bike, the arm, neck, and back muscles mainly work statically when supporting the head and upper body in a sitting position.

The pedaling action, on the other hand, is dynamic muscle work, or more specifically, dynamic–concentric muscle work, which means that the muscle also shortens as it contracts to overcome a load. The opposite, eccentric effort (yielding muscle work), occurs when, for example, landing after jumping off a wall, whereby the hamstrings must work eccentrically; although the muscles do resist, they are stretched (lengthened). The extensor muscles of the leg are vigorously stretched by the eccentric effort phase of the running action (absorption of bodyweight), but they are not at all used to this. This results in microscopic muscle tears (microtrauma), commonly known as "muscle soreness." Triathletes don't suffer from this problem as their leg muscles are accustomed to the eccentric effort by regular running workouts.

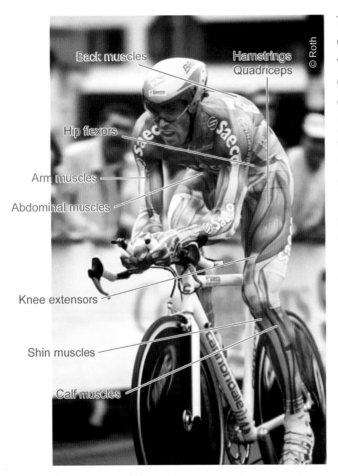

The cyclist's most important muscles are the quadriceps, the size of which is determined by the cyclist's genetic make-up. Racing cyclists do tend to have slim, wiry legs. The hamstrings are used when pulling on the pedals. The pedaling action is supported by the lower leg muscles: the calf assists in the pedaling (both flexion and extension) and the shin muscles help only during the pulling movement, when they hold the feet in position (see chapter 8.2, Smooth Pedal Action).

Fig. 2.1: Blue: working muscles; red: supporting muscles

Bones

The bones in the human body are of lightweight construction, with a solid, external, compact layer encasing the spongy interior. Although they look very stiff and inflexible, bones are actually relatively elastic. Pulling, pushing, bending, and twisting are tolerated to an astonishingly high degree. Cycling is a low-impact sport that is kind to bones and joints, lacking as it does the high impact and compression that are typical of running.

Joints

Joints are formed where cartilage-covered bone ends meet. Usually two, but occasionally three, bones meet to form joints and are connected by tendons, muscles, capsules and ligaments. The cartilage-covered bone ends form the joint surfaces inside the joint. Cartilage is a very pressure-elastic, smooth substance whose durability is as yet unmatched by any man-made substitute.

The joint cavity (space between the ends of the bones) is enclosed by a double-layered capsule, which first provides additional support to the joint and second produces what is known as synovial fluid. A very important joint for the cyclist is the knee joint, a pivotal-hinge joint. The hip joint is also important as it is subject to the constant motion of the femur. The range of motion of the foot joint is relatively low in comparison. The other joints in the body are only moved significantly when changing the sitting position or when pedaling out of the saddle. As cycling is such a low-impact sport, the risk of cartilage damage is low.

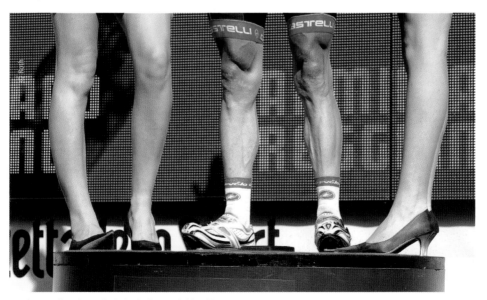

Racing cyclists have little body fat and thin skin.

Cardiovascular system

The physical capacity over endurance performances is predominantly limited by the cardiovascular system, which demonstrates an astonishing ability to adapt to increased demands in an endurance sport such as cycling.

The heart

The blood flowing from the superior and inferior vena cava into the right atrium of the heart from all parts of the body passes through the atrioventricular valves into the ventricle. When the heart contracts, blood is pumped from the right ventricle into the pulmonary artery and enriched with oxygen in the lungs. This oxygen-rich blood flows down the pulmonary veins from the lungs into the left ventricle. This process is known as pulmonary circulation. The left ventricle is filled with the blood in the left atrium, from where it is pumped by a contraction (heart beat) into the aorta, known as systematic circulation. The aorta supplies blood to all organs and structures via multiple exits. The heart valves work to prevent a fatal return flow of blood in the wrong direction. During the contraction phase (systole), blood is ejected, and in the relaxation phase (diastole), it fills with blood again.

The heart rate is subject to a complicated control and regulatory mechanism: the higher the effort, the higher the heart rate, up to a value of about 220 minus age. Cardiac excitation is an automatic process and is not controlled voluntarily; it originates in the sinoatrial node between the two atria and spreads out rhythmically to the rest of the heart from there.

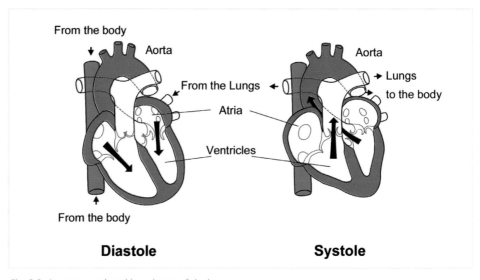

Fig. 2.2: Anatomy and working phases of the heart

An untrained heart weighs between 250 and 300 g, beats about 70 times per minute about 100,000 times per day, in the process circulating 7,000-8,000 l of blood through the body.

Vascular system

Oxygenated blood is circulated through the body via the vascular system, predominantly the arterioles (small arteries) and capillaries. The arterioles and capillaries of the muscles are actively constricted at rest, thereby preventing unnecessary blood flow to the muscles, as the blood is primarily required by the gastro-intestinal tract, kidneys, liver, and brain.

When we start to move, the vessels in the working muscles expand, and more blood, and therefore more oxygen and nutrients, can then flow to the muscle fibers. As a result, circulation in the digestive system is reduced during activity. The muscles require more blood during exercise, so the cardiac pumping capacity increases.

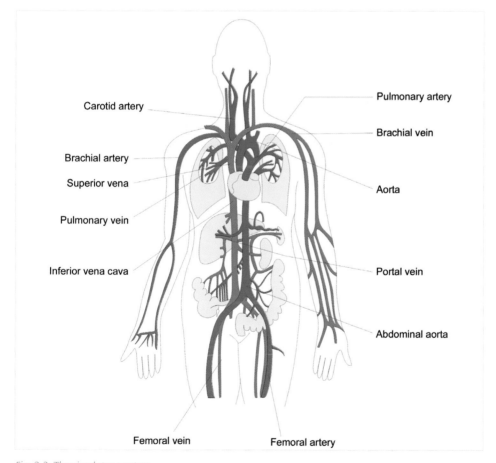

Carotid artery

Pulmonary artery

Brachial vein

Brachial artery

Superior vena

Aorta

Pulmonary vein

Inferior vena cava

Portal vein

Abdominal aorta

Femoral vein   Femoral artery

Fig. 2.3: The circulatory system

The capillaries, the smallest vessels and also the location of gaseous exchanges (oxygen–carbon dioxide, nutrients–metabolites), are connected to the venoles and then the veins. The blood then flows into either the superior or inferior vena cava. The venae cavae then transport the blood back to the heart.

The veins, unlike the arteries, are unable to actively constrict in order to transport blood; however, they do have valves that help the blood to flow back to the heart against the force of gravity. The muscles in the legs, for example, help to pump the blood through the veins to the heart.

Breathing

The right and left lungs are the external respiratory organs. Oxygen-poor, carbon dioxide-rich blood flows into the alveoli, the extremely thin walled capillaries inside the lungs, where the blood releases its carbon dioxide and absorbs oxygen. This process is called *gas exchange* and only takes about 0.3 seconds. With the aid of the breathing muscles, primarily the diaphragm, at rest the lungs expand during inhalation, air flows down the trachea and bronchia into the pulmonary alveoli where the gas exchange takes place, and finally the carbon dioxide air escapes from the lungs (exhalation). The lungs are very elastic. They work like a balloon: They inflate during inhalation, and they deflate during exhalation. Only during exercise (e.g., cycling) when breathing is heavier is the diaphragm supported by chest breathing. A whole series of auxiliary respiratory muscles then reinforce the inhalation and exhalation processes and increase the energy requirement of the respiratory muscles up to 10% of the total energy requirement. Specific respiratory muscle training can increase the efficiency of these muscles, which decreases their oxygen and energy consumption. For each breath at rest, only about 0.5 l of air is breathed in and out 15 times per minute (=7.5 l); while at maximum effort, the trained mountain biker may inhale and exhale over 190 l of air per minute after a finishing sprint, for example.

The *vital capacity*–the maximum amount of air that a person can expel from the lungs after first filling the lungs to their maximum–is highly dependent on age, gender, and body size. The vital capacity is usually between three and seven liters, but it reveals little about a mountain biker's absolute endurance ability. The elite African distance runners, for example, have small lungs compared to Europeans but still usually run faster.

As previously mentioned, the gas exchange in the lungs is termed *external respiration*, while the metabolism (i.e., combustion in the cells) is called *internal respiration*.

Organ Systems

Nervous system

Every single physical process and action is governed by the nervous system, partly consciously and partly unconsciously. The nervous system senses, processes, and reacts to stimuli with the aid of the sensory and effector organs that enable us to interact with the world. The nervous system consists of many milliards of cells that have lost the ability to divide.

From an anatomical point of view, we distinguish between the central nervous system (CNS: brain and spinal cord) and the peripheral nervous system (PNS) with the nerves that represent the connection to the sensory and effector organs. From a functional point of view, we differentiate between the voluntary (somatic) and involuntary (autonomic) nervous systems. The somatic nervous system carries all voluntary movement commands to the corresponding effector organs, usually muscles.

While the brain constitutes the control center of the nervous system, the spinal cord is the wiring system responsible for transferring information to and from the effector organs along the nerves that run down the spinal cord protected by the vertebrae. Secondly, like the brain, the spinal cord is the nerve center for subordinate processes, such as the reflexes.

The autonomic nervous system, which controls all unconscious processes in the body, consists of two different sub-systems which have completely different areas of activity. The parasympathetic nervous system is responsible for all physical functions at rest (digestion, recovery). The sympathetic nervous system, on the other hand, controls physical activity and boosts the mobilization of the organ system responsible for movement.

Digestion

In the following example, a cyclist who has eaten a muesli bar illustrates the digestive process from ingestion to excretion. The times given are a rough guide only and may differ considerably depending on circumstances.

3:30pm: A test cyclist starts a three- to four-hour training ride. His last meal was not a big one, eaten three hours previously.

5:00pm: The cyclist eats a muesli bar. He breaks it down mechanically using his teeth, and his saliva turns it into a slippery pulp (bolus or chyme). 1 Saliva enzymes in the mouth already start to break down the complex carbohydrates.

5:01pm: The muesli bolus travels down the esophagus (gullet) to the stomach. Peristalsis (muscle contractions) helps to accelerate it down the 30-cm long esophagus. **2**

5:02pm: Now in the stomach, the muesli bar triggers the production of hydrochloric acid and enzymes, which process the bolus chemically into gastric juice. **3** Roughly 1.5-2 l of gastric juice are produced daily. Only fats and proteins are attacked by the enzymes, while the carbohydrates are not broken down any further here. The hydrochloric acid continues to break down the rough muesli bolus.

5:03pm: Water secretion dilutes the chyme, which is mixed up thoroughly like a cement mixer by the movements of the stomach walls. At fast cycling speeds, the body wastes no energy on digestion, and the digestive process is postponed until a more gentle stage of the ride.

5:09pm: The stomach continues to work like a mixer; slowly the fats rise to the surface of the chyme while the carbohydrates are deposited on the stomach fundus.

5:25pm: The chyme is further diluted and now only takes a few minutes to leave the stomach. High-carbohydrate drinks would already be in the intestine by now.

5:40pm: Finally, just before the cyclist hits the "wall," the stomach opens its pyloric sphincter at its lower end and allows the chyme to gradually enter the duodenum. The pancreas secretes enzymes to break down carbohydrates, proteins, and fats into the duodenum, and the secretion of bile acid for fat digestion also starts.

5:43pm: Rhythmic (peristaltic) movements push the muesli bar into the adjacent small intestine. The complex carbohydrates broken down into glucose are now absorbed into the blood through the villi that protrude from the lining of the intestine and make their way toward the liver via the portal vein system. Part of the fat has already been broken down into fatty acids and glycerin; also the proteins have, in the meantime, been broken down into individual amino acids. Their absorption (resorption) starts gradually.

5:46pm: The chyme travels farther down the small intestine, the top third of which mainly serves to absorb glucose. **4** The glucose travels to the liver via the portal vein system, where the glucose molecules are turned into glycogen. Some of the glycogen is stored in the liver (size of the deposit: 100-130 g glycogen), while the rest travels to the muscles where it is either stored or burned immediately. Also the amino acids, fatty acids, and vitamins A, B, C, E, and K as well as the minerals are absorbed into the blood from the small intestine.

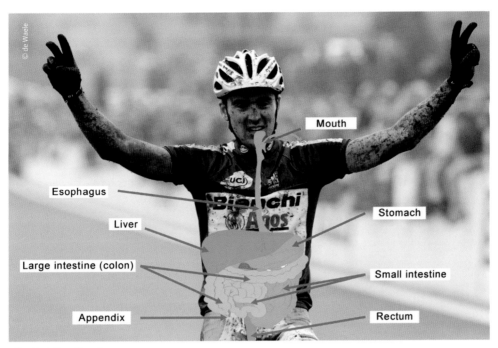

Fig. 2.4: The digestive system

6:30pm: Remains of the muesli can still be found in the small intestine.

7:00pm: End of the training ride. Almost all of the glucose has now been resorbed, and the proteins have also been partially absorbed. Fat digestion and resorption takes a while longer.

7:30pm: The process starts again as the cyclist eats his evening meal. The amino acids from the bar have now reached the liver, where they are reassembled into proteins—known as plasma protein—and travel into the blood. Excess protein (in the case of excessive calorie consumption or lack of food) is burned off or converted into fat and stored (see chapter 5).

10:30pm: The rest of the muesli bar leaves the small intestine for the rectum. 5 80- 90% of the nutrients have now been removed from the chyme. In the colon, the water used for digestion must be removed. This means that the consistency of the chyme becomes thicker and drier as it passes through the colon. At the top of the colon, more minerals and remaining nutrients are absorbed.

The next morning: The muesli bar leaves the body in the form of feces. Fatty foods would take about 10 hours longer to digest.

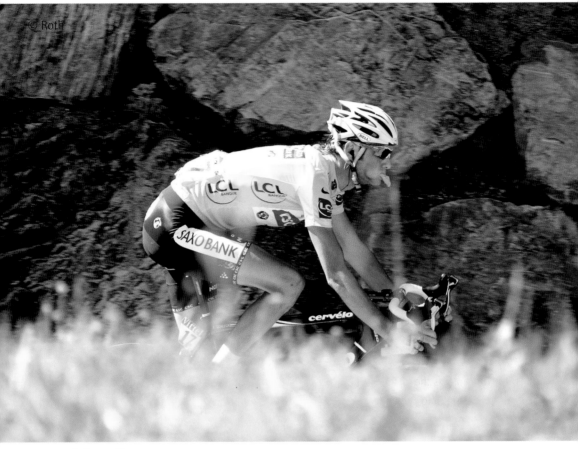

Eating on the go

Kidneys

The kidneys play a very important role in the body as blood filters and excretory organs. In the case of cycling they have to work overtime, as their filtering action has to keep pace with the increased calorie burning associated with physical exercise. Salts, metabolites of the protein metabolism process, water, and also foreign substances are eliminated from the blood and therefore from the body by the kidneys. From the 1,500 l blood that flow through the kidneys on a daily basis, about 150 l of primary urine is filtered, which eventually is concentrated into about 1.5 l of urine and eliminated.

Blood

The 5-6 liters of blood in our bodies consists of roughly 55% blood plasma (fluid) and about 45% of various blood cells. Blood accounts for about 5-6% of our bodyweight. Endurance training, such as mountain biking, increases blood volume by about 15%.

These are the main functions attributed to blood:

- transport (oxygen, carbon dioxide, nutrients, metabolic waste, hormones)
- heat circulation and transportation
- clotting
- immune defense

A couple of interesting facts about blood: 1 mm^3 of blood (i.e., a tiny amount) contains an incredible 4.5-5 million red blood corpuscles and about 5,000-8,000 white blood corpuscles for immune defense; 100 ml of blood also contains about 7 g of protein. The red blood corpuscles (erythrocytes) are responsible for transporting oxygen and carbon dioxide.

2.2   Performance Physiology

Effects of training on the heart, circulation, and muscles
This section explains the changes in the heart, circulation, and muscles that take place during the endurance training process (cycling). Terms like *sports heart*, *resting heart rate* and *maximal oxygen uptake* (**VO$_2$max**) are explained in detail.

Two adaptation phases
The adaptation process of the body is split into two phases: *functional and dimensional*. At low training volumes and intensities in recreational and leisure cycling, the adaptation is purely *functional*, characterized by an improvement in muscle metabolism, leading to a more efficient cardiovascular system. This increased efficiency is due to lowered circulation. In other words, the resting heart rate and exercise heart rate are slightly lowered. The second phase of adaptation is *dimensional* adaptation in which the dimensions (sizes) of the organs change.

A bigger engine
Regular, long-term endurance training leads to an adaptation process in the heart that results in what is known as *athlete's heart*. Athlete's heart is characterized by an increase in size and concomitant drop in heart rate. This adaptation process is a result of the faster metabolism, especially in the muscles whose increased oxygen and nutritional requirements can only be met by greater blood circulation, which in turn requires a more efficient heart.

While an untrained heart weighs about 300 g, that of an endurance athlete can weigh up to 500 g. This increase in weight is accompanied by an increase in size. From about 800 ml for men and 500 ml for women, heart size can increase up to 900-1200 ml, and in rare cases up to 1,500 ml. The largest hearts can be found in road-racing cyclists and are the result of their often extreme endurance training loads.

The increase in heart volume enables a greater stroke volume. *The stroke volume* is the amount of blood that the heart pumps into the aorta per beat (80 ml for the untrained athlete and up to 150 ml for trained endurance athletes). However, as the body does not need more blood for the same performance, the heart can pump more slowly. The maximum possible *cardiac output per minute*, or the total amount of blood pumped by the left side of the heart per minute (heart rate x stroke volume; e.g., 70 x 80 ml = 5.6 l/min at rest), rises compared to an untrained person so that the muscles have more blood available to them per unit of time.

Lower revs

The maximum heart rate increases only minimally after years of endurance training so that the greater maximum stroke volume produces a greatly increased maximum cardiac output per minute. At maximum effort, the untrained individual attains a cardiac output of about 20 l, while someone with endurance training can attain values of over 30 l.

A clear indicator of athlete's heart is a lowered heart rate from about 60-70 bpm (70-80 for women) for an untrained person to 40-50 bpm at high-performance level. At pro level, resting heart rates of below 40 bpm are common and may occasionally be as low as 30. The lowering of resting heart rate in recreational and leisure cyclists to 50-60 bpm is not usually caused by increased heart size, but, as already mentioned, is caused by a transfer and calming of the vegetative nervous system. Training should never just stop completely once your active cycling career is over, as this can cause the heart to suffer potentially dangerous training withdrawal symptoms.

The advantages of athlete's heart:
- greater efficiency
- the same performance can be achieved with a lower heart rate
- lower resting and working heart rate, which protects the heart (comparable to lower revs in a car)
- efficient circulatory system
- other positive physical adaptation processes that take place during the development of athlete's heart

Maximum oxygen uptake

Maximum oxygen uptake (**VO$_2$max**) is a very important physiological measurement in cycling, as it is the key criterium for endurance ability.

VO$_2$max is the greatest possible amount of oxygen—not breath—that the mountain biker can inhale under maximum loading conditions via his lungs into his blood. The way to measure the **VO$_2$max** accurately is on an exercise bike as part of a performance test. The normal value for an untrained person is roughly 3 l oxygen per minute and can be increased by appropriate training to 5-6 l per minute.

The **VO$_2$max** depends on the athlete's fitness, age, sex, and weight. For example, a heavier person will need more oxygen for the same external performance than a lighter person, because he has more bodyweight to move. For this reason, the weight-related **VO$_2$max** is used in order to obtain an accurate measurement of performance potential and to compare different athletes. The weight-related or relative **VO$_2$max** gives the oxygen intake per kilogram bodyweight and minute.

The pros can attain values between 80-90 ml oxygen per min and kg bodyweight; untrained cyclists 20 to 30 years old, on the other hand, only reach 40-45 ml per kg bodyweight and min. The maximum oxygen intake for an untrained male declines by 1% per year, while women only lose 0.8%per year. However, most sedentary individuals do not know that this process can be stopped and even reversed by endurance training. A fit 70-year-old can still attain the same results as an untrained 30-year-old. Factors that influence **VO$_2$max** (as well as age, weight, and sex) are:

- the circulation transporting capacity (cardiac output),
- the oxygen transporting capacity of the blood,
- respiration and gas exchange in the lungs,
- blood supply to the muscles (capillarization), and
- intramuscular metabolism (enzyme loading).

Muscles

Training allows human muscle mass to be doubled, even tripled. Our muscles contain slow-twitch (type I) and fast-twitch (type II) fibers, as well as a hybrid type (intermediate fibers). The intermediate, medium-fast fibers have the ability to turn into fast twitch fibers. The slow, or red fibers, are the endurance fibers. These fibers are predominately in cyclists, with the exception of track cyclists (70-90%; even up to 95% in top cyclists). The fast, or white, muscle fibers are thicker, tire more quickly, and are mainly found in speed-strength and strength athletes. The proportions are almost reversed; up to 80% belong to the fast fiber type. The proportion of fibers in untrained individuals varies depending on their body type, and the limits can be shifted to a certain extent by training. The process by which white fibers are converted to red or vice versa is still not fully understood, but it is clear that the type of exercise performed (endurance or strength) is probably what triggers the change. The latest research shows that it is easier to convert fast-twitch fibers to slow-twitch than the other way around. As it is not yet clear whether the transformation is also possible in the opposite direction, it must be assumed that world-class endurance athletes are born with an extremely high proportion of slow-twitch fibers.

However, it is considerably easier to reach a good endurance level through training than a good sprinting level. Among road-cycling pros, only a handful of cyclists possess a combination of both excellent endurance and sprinting ability, such as Erik Zabel.

As the thinner, red muscle fibers, surrounded by many capillaries, are beneficial for the aerobic metabolism, the road cyclist should not aim to build as much muscle mass as possible (see chapter 3.8, Strength Training). The additional muscle mass would also need to be supplied with oxygen.

Endurance training improves the capillarization (the amount of capillaries per muscle fiber) of the muscle tissue, which means that the metabolic and gas exchange surfaces between the muscle fibers and the blood increase in size, thus enabling the metabolism to work faster and more efficiently.

Metabolism

There are three types of energy supply available to the muscles, which are shown here in isolation for the sake of clarity but are actually all interconnected like cogs. The transitions from one type of energy supply to another are fluid. The types concerned are the aerobic energy supply and the anaerobic energy supply, which is further divided into the anaerobic—alactic and the anaerobic—lactic acid energy supply.

Aerobic energy supply

Aerobic means that energy is released with the aid of oxygen. In cycling, the aerobic energy supply is the most important metabolic pathway, as it can work for long periods of time, can provide relatively high amounts of energy, and can refill and regenerate both anaerobic metabolic pathways after they have been exhausted. In the aerobic metabolism, fats and carbohydrates are burned or oxidized.

The most important fuel is glucose (aerobic glycolysis), a simple carbohydrate with the chemical formula $C_6H_{12}O_6$. Glucose is the degradation product of the complex carbohydrates (see chapter 5). To greatly simplify the process, the glucose combines with oxygen and is split into carbon dioxide (exhaled from the lungs) and water. A relatively large amount of energy in the form of ATP (adenosine triphosphate, a very energy-rich molecule) is released in the process. ATP is the direct energy store of the cells and is used as muscle fuel that ultimately triggers muscle contraction. The complexity of the individual reaction stages from glucose to ATP exceeds the scope of this book.

Steam Engine

In a very basic way, the energy supply system can be compared to a steam engine.

The fuels (fats and glucose) represent water; the fire, sometimes smaller, sometimes larger, represents the metabolic pathway. The steam, made of water, represents the ATP. In order to move or propel something forward, the cell requires ATP, just as the steam engine requires steam. As the body's ATP store is limited, so is the steam store in the boiler, meaning that it must constantly be stoked.

Aerobic energy is produced in the muscle fibers, specifically, the mitochondria. The *mitochondrion* is termed the *powerhouse* of the cells. Glucose is either extracted by the blood and broken down or it comes from the glycogen stores in the cells (glycogen is the storage form of glucose), from which it is transported to the mitochondria.

As well as carbohydrates, fats are also burned on the aerobic pathway. Fats are composed of fatty acids, which enter the carbohydrate metabolism and are burned together with the carbohydrates. For this reason, energy can only be obtained from fats when carbohydrates are being burned. The disadvantage of fat-burning is that it only occurs at very low exercise intensities due to the high oxygen requirement.

However, the stored amount of energy or calorific value is twice as high as that of carbohydrates (9.3 kcal compared to 4.1 kcal per g).

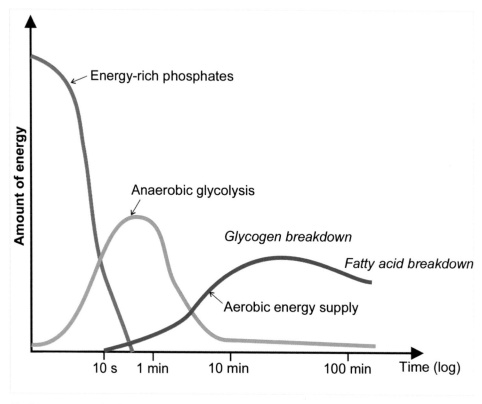

Fig. 2.5: Energy supply related to exercise duration

The cyclist's fat metabolism must be trained in order to maintain the highly performance-limiting glycogen stores, which are completely emptied after about two hours of intensive effort. While the untrained individual can use roughly 40% of the energy required for fat metabolism, the trained endurance athlete can use 60% and above. With increasing endurance fitness, the proportion of fat used to provide energy increases at the same intensity. This protects the precious glycogen reserves so that they are still available for race-deciding, high-intensity bursts. The endurance-trained cyclist can therefore store two to three times more fat for energy production in the muscle cells than the untrained individual.

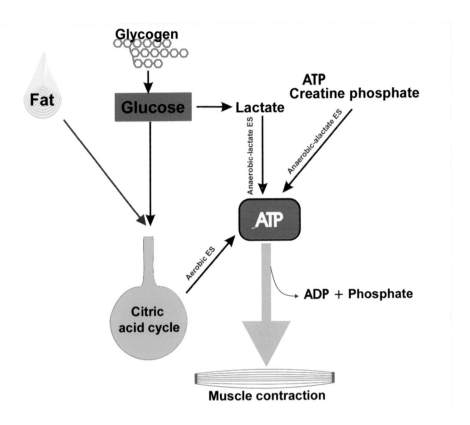

Fig. 2.6: Simplified diagram of the energy metabolism

Glycogen: Limited Stock

If a cyclist's basic endurance is not well-developed, the muscle cells already start to draw on the glycogen at relatively low training loads. Between 400 and 500 g of glycogen are stored in the liver and muscles, with the majority being in the muscles. The amount of stored muscle glycogen is critical when it comes to cycling performance. If the glycogen reserves are empty after the race, they must be refilled, which takes between 24 and 48 hours even with an optimum diet (see chapter 5 on nutrition). Endurance training improves the metabolism in the muscle fibers. The enzyme content in the mitochondria in trained endurance cyclists is higher and the substrates (glucose, fatty acids) exist in higher concentrations ready to be broken down than in the untrained cyclist.

The number of mitochondria per muscle fiber also increases and oxygen can be used more easily and in greater amounts thanks to improved capillarization (number of capillaries per muscle fiber). The aerobic metabolism of the trained cyclist is faster and more efficient due to this.

Anaerobic energy supply

Anaerobic–Lactic Acid Energy Supply

Anaerobic means energy supply without using oxygen. On this metabolic pathway, lactate, or lactic acid, is produced, hence the name lactic acid energy supply. Lactate causes hyperacidity of the muscles and makes the legs feel heavy, forcing you to stop. The muscles always use the lactic formation metabolic pathway when the required performance cannot be achieved by aerobic combustion alone.

In the cells, glucose is split into lactate in the absence of oxygen. This continues until the glycolytic enzyme (responsible for the splitting) is blocked by the hyperacidity caused by the lactate and stops working. At this splitting of glucose, energy is again released in the form of ATP. However, it is amazing that the anaerobic splitting of a glucose molecule only provides about

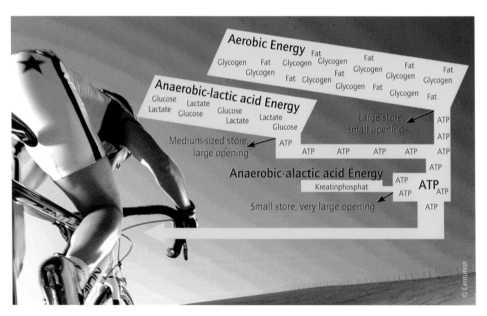

Fig. 2.7: The energy stores in the human body (simplified). The types of energy supply are interconnected. The large stock of aerobic energy can only be used slowly; for larger amounts of energy, the anaerobic–lactic acid store is used, although this is quickly depleted. Short (a few seconds) movements with very high energy consumption use the anaerobic–alactic stores (creatine phosphate). All three pathways create ATP, which is split into ADP for muscle contraction. The stores refill the ATP pool again.

5% of the combustion energy of the aerobic pathway, but also blocks the lactic acid energy supply, managing to supply a higher amount of energy per unit of time. This is because, theoretically, an unlimited number of glucose molecules can be split at the same time, and their total energy is able to ensure a very high performance output for a relatively short time of 40-60 seconds.

At the start of a ride, particularly a race, the aerobic energy supply is not yet running optimally, especially if the warm-up was inadequate. In this case, going into oxygen debt enables the energy deficit to be covered by the anaerobic–lactic acid pathway. The resulting lactic acid is called warm-up lactate, and it is burned away once the aerobic metabolism kicks in. Lactate also builds up during intermediate sprints or attacks. However, if the lactate production exceeds a certain concentration that is so high that it blocks the other metabolic pathways, the lactate can no longer be burned on the aerobic pathway. Then the rider will be forced to drop out due to muscle hyperacidity.

Two cycling disciplines are prime examples of anaerobic–lactic acid energy supply: the 1,000-m time trial and track sprints. Also in road cycling in short circuit time trials up to 1,500 m, there is complete exhaustion of the energy supply under lactate production. These disciplines demand maximum effort in a very short period of time for which aerobic combustion is both too slow and also unable to provide the required amount of energy.

Anaerobic–Alactic Acid Energy Supply

The anaerobic–alactic energy supply is mentioned only for the sake of completeness, as it only plays a subordinate role in cycling. It is vital for strength athletes like weight-lifters, shot-putters, and also for those who practice jumping events. Alactic means that, unlike the anaerobic–lactic acid energy supply, no lactate is created.

The ATP and creatine phosphate reserves (energy-rich phosphate compound) are used up during this energy supply in a maximum of 5-8 seconds, which unfortunately suffices for only a few maximal muscle contractions. It is important to understand that ATP is essential for every muscle contraction; without ATP the muscle cannot contract. For this reason, the cells' ATP reserves must constantly be replenished, predominantly on the aerobic metabolic pathway. ATP is also necessary for other energy-consuming processes in the cells, such as recovery processes or cell growth. When a phosphate residue is split off from ATP, the stored energy is released and the muscle contracts. The remaining ADP (adenosine diphosphate) is later "recycled" into ATP when a phosphate residue is split from creatine phosphate.

Physical adaptations due to regular cycling training (endurance training)

Muscles
↑	Higher performance capacity
↑	Increased capillarization
↑	Larger glycogen stores
↑	More mitochondria

Heart
↑	Greater volume
↑	Increased weight
↑	Greater maximal heart rate
↓	Lower resting heart rate
↓	Lower heart rate during constant exercise

Blood
↑	Greater volume
↑	Better flow characteristics
↑	Increased oxygen transport capacity

Lungs
↑	Increased volume
↑	Increased VO_2max
↓	Lower breathing rate

Body
↑	Increased metabolic efficiency
↑	Strengthened immune system
↑	Greater performance capacity
↓	Reduced fatiguability
↓	Reduced bodyweight

2.3 Cycling Discipline Demand Profiles

The characteristic physiological demands for each race type are listed next. The different endurance zones are explained in chapter 3.1

1. Cycle tours

These races place varying demands on the cyclist, ranging from a race simulation over a time trial to a relaxed training ride in the basic endurance zone, and course distances can vary from 40-200 km (25-124 mi), depending on the cyclist's fitness and objectives. Such a wide range makes it impossible to give a specific demand profile so that the interested reader can evaluate himself and take a look at the corresponding race type (distance) that most closely matches his cycle tour.

2. Road races from 60-120 km

At amateur level, road races are limited to distances up to 120 km (100 mi), although all road races for youth cyclists, juniors, and women fall into this category. Because of the wide time range covered by the long endurance III category (90 min-6 hr) (see chapter 3), these races, as do most amateur circuit races, fall into this category. As in all races, it is possible for the cyclist to ride in the slipstream, thereby reducing the effort intensity. The proportion of anaerobic energy supply can be as high as 10% in shorter races. The exhaustion of the VO_2max in shorter races may occasionally be as high as 95%. The heart rate zone is around 150-195 bpm, although a little higher for youth and juniors due to their higher maximal pulse rate.

3. Road races from 120-200 km

Road races over these distances last 3-6 hours and therefore fall into the long endurance III category (see chapter 3). For such distances, strength must be very well rationed and reserved for decisive race situations (e.g., attacks, climbs, and sprints); 95% and more of the energy supply is covered by the aerobic pathway by the oxidation of fats and carbohydrates. The anaerobic energy supply is less than 5%. The heart rate ranges from 140-180 bpm, sometimes even higher (up to 195 bpm). Performance capacity is primarily determined by the VO_2max value, approximately 60-90% of which is solicited during the race. It is absolutely vital to eat and drink due to the high demands placed on the glycogen stores (about 80% are used up) and increasing dehydration.

4. Circuit races and criteriums over 40-60 km

Circuit races in the youth, junior, and women's categories are mainly held over these distances. The exercise intensity is very high, at 80-95% VO_2max. The heart rate lies in the region of

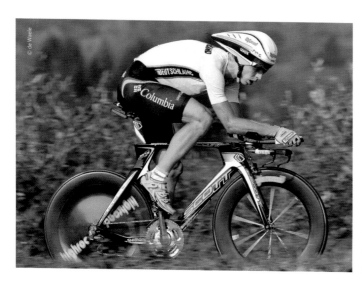

Motivation and equipment are key factors in time trials.

170-195 bpm and is slightly higher for the youth cyclists. Around 90% of the energy is covered by the aerobic metabolism, and 10% is covered anaerobically. Their competitive nature and frequent sprints require a very dynamic riding style characterized by many changes of pace. Intermediate sprints and numerous attacks at any point of the race mean cyclists require very high speed and strength levels coupled with a well-developed aerobic capacity. The cadence in circuit races is usually higher than in road races. If the pre-race diet has been good, eating during the race is less important, although it is still essential to drink, even during short races, in order to maintain performance levels (see chapter 5).

5. Circuit races and criteriums from 60-100 km

Circuit races over 60-100 km (37-62 mi) also fall into the long endurance III category and are usually only contested by amateurs. They are characterized by abrupt changes of race situation. The demands on the cyclist vary greatly according to his ability, so that for example a rider in the pack may ride a less intensive race than one in the lead or in breakaway groups. The frequent curves, up to 320 in 80 km, place high demands on the muscles as each one requires a brief burst of anaerobic energy.

6. Stage races

Stage races are the hardest the sport has to offer, apart from the newly fashionable extreme endurance races such as the triple ultra-triathlon. The individual races are usually long endurance III, with all the associated demands. To be able to reproduce such performances over several days, sometimes even over several weeks (the Tour de France lasts for three weeks), is an excellent example of the extreme endurance trainability of the human body.

As the daily energy requirement often exceeds what a person can consume in food form, the metabolism reaches its limit, and it is not uncommon for muscle protein as well as body fat to be broken down during a stage race.

7. Individual time trials

Individual time trials lack a tactical aspect, as success is determined only by the actual performance capacity. Individual time trials are held over a wide range of distances, which makes it quite difficult to provide typical physiological features. Short time trials lasting less than 10 minutes place an almost maximal load on the cardiovascular system. The heart rate is submaximal to maximal at 190-210 bpm.

The oxygen uptake is almost maximal and the anaerobic energy supply can reach 20%. This is why hyperacidification (high lactate concentration) in short time trials is very high. The longer the time trial distance, the closer it approaches long endurance category II. Time trials are usually characterized by a very even distribution of effort, and the heart rate is also regular.

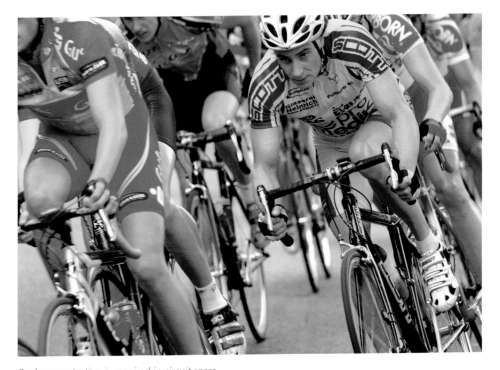

Peak concentration is required in circuit races.

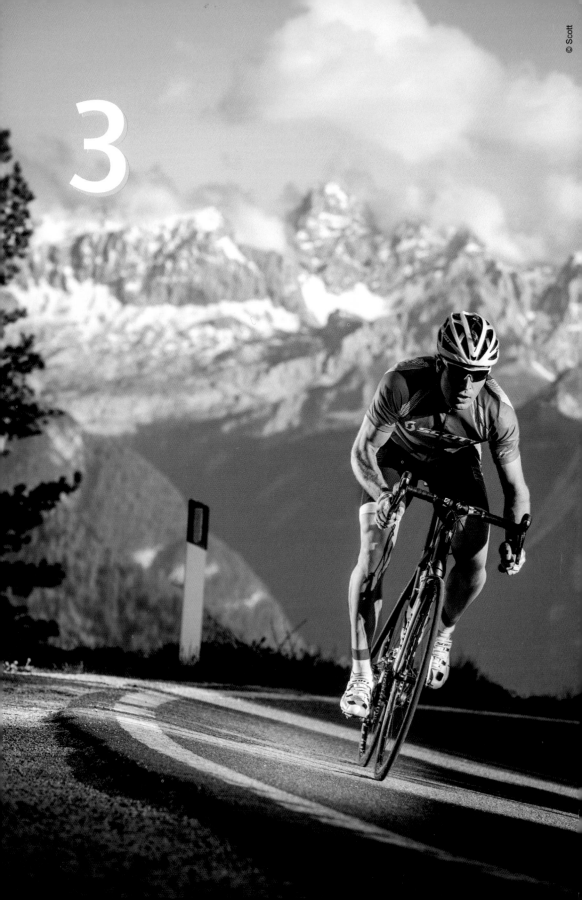

3

3   Training

3.1   Basic Principles of Training Theory

Training theory is the study of the theory and practice of athletic training and plays an important role in sports science. It mainly involves choosing the right training form in order to optimize the training process.

Training is, or should be, a planned activity; the "should" indicates that in cycling, as in other sports, this is often not the case. Even though the tendency in recent years has increasingly been to stick to a planned training program, the fact is that training is often ill-thought out and aimless, wasting time that would lead to much better performances if training were more structured.

In order to train intelligently and to understand training plans, it is first necessary to understand the basic principles of training theory so that it can then be put into practice in your everyday training. Even though top cyclists do not need to worry about drawing up training plans, background information is very valuable when it comes to understanding the planned workout and, if necessary, changing it should it prove unsuitable. Likewise, hobby cyclists can also

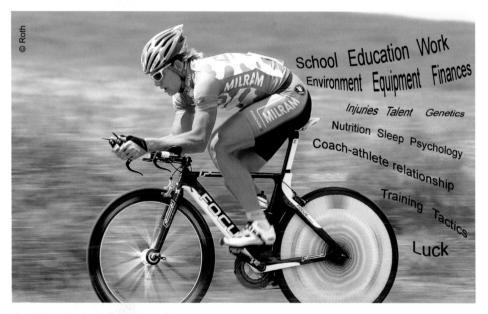

Fig. 3.1: Performance factors in cycling

manage and track their performance development. However, the importance of this knowledge is still very often underestimated. Exercise testing and prescription as it relates to cycling as an endurance sport are explained generally in the following sections.

Definition

Training, as mentioned earlier, is a planned process that aims to improve or maintain athletic performance using appropriate training methods. Athletic performance not only means purely physical athletic ability, but also includes tactical, technical, and mental aspects.

From a biological point of view, training is the body's reaction to exercise. When the human body exercises, physical abilities improve, but if that exercise ceases, these abilities disappear (use it or lose it!). The correct sequencing of training and rest is crucial for training to be effective. Training disturbs the body's biological equilibrium, so that after the rest phase, the body adapts to the training load and achieves a higher performance level than before.

Supercompensation

The following diagram illustrates the principle of *supercompensation*, one of the most important principles of training theory. Training stimulus, fatigue, recovery, and supercompensation must follow each other in this order, with the correct time intervals between them.

Recovery is the process by which the body recuperates from fatigue and lasts until the previous performance level has been regained.

Supercompensation is the term given to the performance improvement following recovery; it is a kind of "over-recovery." The improved performance level is achieved because recovery does not stop when the previous performance level has been reached, but continues until a performance level has been reached that can easily cope with the same training load on the next occasion. This process is known as *adaptation*.

Once a high training level has been achieved, improvements in performance level become smaller until eventually there is a constant performance level plateau. This is why very fit cyclists need very high training volumes and sophisticated training plans to maintain or, if possible, improve their performance level, as constantly increasing training loads alone is not sufficient to be able to perform at elite level. For more on physiological adaptation processes, see chapter 2.2.

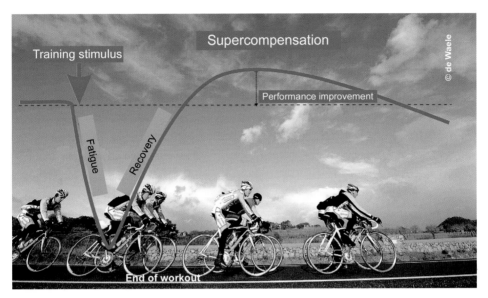

Fig. 3.2: The principle of supercompensation

Describing training
Training intensity
Means the extent of the workload from a loading stimulus or training session. The easiest way to establish training intensity in mountain biking is by measuring the heart rate (high intensity = high heart rate). Other intensity indicators are lactate concentration or speed.

Training volume
Is the total of all loading or training stimuli performed per training session or training period (week, preparation phase). In cycling, training volume can be compared to training mileage (e.g., 100 km per day or 400 km per week) or better still by the training duration. Training sessions without the bike (e.g., gym training, exercises, running training, strength training) should also be included when calculating training volume.

Training density
Gives the relationship between training and rest (recovery) and also the rest duration between the individual training stimuli, while also differentiating between complete and incomplete rest. *Complete rest* means waiting until the body has completely recovered before resuming training. This again can be measured by heart rate or by how your body feels. *Incomplete rest* means resuming training when the heart rate returns to levels of 120-130 bpm, at which point training is resumed.

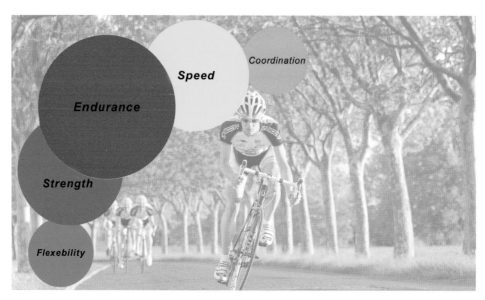

Fig. 3.3: Components of fitness

Training duration
Is the length of a bout of training, such as an interval (3 min) or a series of sprints (6 x 20 sec).

Training frequency
Means how many times per week training takes place. In cycling, training should not take place less than four times per week, and if necessary due to time constraints, two sessions may be performed in one day (e.g., before and after work or an event) and may increase to over 10. Good amateurs usually train six or seven times per week (including running).

These five basic training factors enable accurate descriptions of the training process and are used next.

As already mentioned, training involves alternating between activity and rest, thus raising the issues of optimal training dosing and sequencing. The recovery phase is considered to be the most important, because this is when performance improvement takes place; the training itself only serves to trigger recovery and subsequent supercompensation. Excessively intensive training and inadequate recovery are the main reasons why many cyclists fail to improve despite training for long periods. If the body is constantly exercised hard and is not given time to recover between workouts, it is being trained into the ground, meaning that performance level drops in spite of all the hard work. However, if training stimuli are set correctly, performance levels will increase up to an *individual performance limit*, which in an endurance sport like cycling can only be reached after many years of training. It is therefore impossible to reach elite level in cycling in just a few years if you have not previously practiced an endurance sport. This fact is often hard to understand and a source of frustration for newcomers to the sport.

Right and wrong!

The following graph shows a training sequence that is too short; training resumes before the recovery process is over, thus making it impossible for the performance level to improve and even causes it to dip.

Performance stagnation would be the result of training too infrequently (i.e., when training is resumed only after the supercompensation is over, when the condition of the body is almost the same as before training). This results in little or no training progress. *Figure 3.4* shows that training must resume right in the middle (high point) of the supercompensation phase for optimal performance improvement. As well as the recovery lengths between the training sessions, the training and racing themselves must be right for performance to improve; more on this in the next chapter. If the training workload is too low, the adaptation process will not be

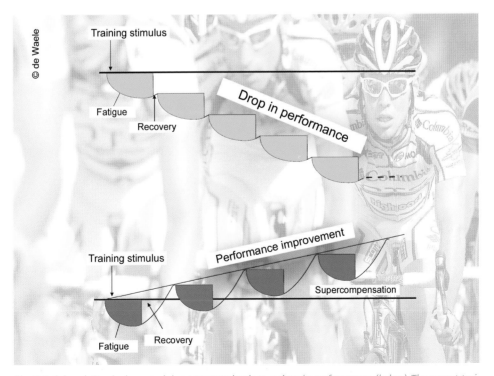

Fig. 3.4: (above) Overly dense training sequence leads to a drop in performance. (below) The correct training stimuli performed in the supercompensation phase leads to the desired performance improvement.

triggered, while too much training in the long term leads to overtraining. Only the correct training will cause the desired adaptation and supercompensation. *Correct training* means that training type, volume, and intensity and the rest phases must all be perfectly aligned.

Awareness of your own body must also be taken into account when determining rest phases and drawing up a training plan in general. Suggested training plans, like those in this book, must be adapted to individual circumstances. A training plan should not be viewed as being set in stone.

Recovery
What determines the duration of the recovery phase?
A basic principle of recovery states that the harder or more exhausting the training or race, the longer the body will take to recover, because the body needs longer to compensate for the disruption, or biological imbalance, caused to its tissues. Illnesses like infections or inflammations usually delay recovery. Daily workouts then become harder to cope with and the recovery phase takes longer. After heavy head colds, recovery can be affected for two to three weeks, thus significantly affecting performance levels. Stress and other psychological factors can also negatively impact the ability to recover. Recovery duration varies from one person to another; one cyclist is capable of putting in another peak performance the very next day after a hard race, while another may only be fit again three days or even a week later. This helps to explain why some cyclists can only produce good performances in one-day races and in circuits, which only allow for short recovery times; they are not able to cope.

How is recovery affected?
Recovery is only affected when post-training and racing preconditions are optimal, but there is no "miracle method" that enables immediate recovery. What prerequisites should be kept in mind?

Factors that enhance recovery:

- Sufficient rest (sleep)
- Recovery nutrition
- Stretching
- Massage
- Warm bath
- Recovery training

Sufficient rest does not just mean avoiding unnecessary effort after exercise, but it also inclu-des getting sufficient bed rest. The diet must be very high in carbohydrates, vitamins, and mi-nerals in order to replenish the empty energy reserves (see chapter 5). Stretching lowers muscle tone, maintains flexibility, and, combined with a massage, a warm bath, and recovery training, accelerates the elimination of metabolites.

However, the best way to accelerate recovery is endurance training; well-trained cyclists are usually relatively fresh and recovered a few minutes after finishing an exhausting race, while beginners may even find it hard to recover from a mountain section to the extent that they are even forced to drop out of the race or training ride.

Adaptation

In the **adaptation** process, metabolic adaptation is limited by *morphological* adaptation (phy-sical adaptation; e.g., muscles, heart). An endurance sport like cycling causes significant adap-tation processes, both metabolic and morphological, as described in more detail in chapter 2.2.

Theoretical principles of endurance

Endurance in general means the body's increased ability to withstand fatigue and to recover afterward (resistance to fatigue, both physical and mental). As already mentioned, endurance is one of the factors of conditioning, but not the only important one for cycling, as strength and speed are also necessary for good performances. Strength in particular has been badly neglected for decades, and it is only in the last 15 years that training science has started to recognize the importance of strength for all sports (see chapter 3.8).

There are several different forms of endurance training, not all of which are relevant for cy-cling; however, for the sake of completeness they are presented here: local endurance is the opposite of general endurance; local endurance is limited to less than 1/6 of all muscles. In cycling, the use of large muscles groups (the legs) corresponds to general endurance. Depen-ding on the type of metabolism involved, we distinguish between aerobic (sufficient oxygen present) and anaerobic endurance (too little oxygen present); both aerobic and anaerobic endurance are required in cycling. There is yet another difference between static (static endu-rance without movement) and dynamic endurance (movement). However, the most important difference for cycling is based on exercise duration, which may last from 35 seconds to more than 6 hours.

Different types of endurance

1   Short-term endurance (35 sec-2 min)

Short-term endurance is characterized by a high metabolic rate per unit of time. In cycling there are very few disciplines that fall into this category (e.g., the 500- and 1,000-m time trials on the track and extremely short circuit time trials contested by amateurs). A premature spurt in sprint disciplines on the track are also classified as short-term endurance. Lactate values of up to 20 mmol/l blood may be attained (e.g., in 1,000-m time trials), values that would immediately put a road cyclist into a coma. About 60% of the energy is supplied anaerobically.

The following prerequisites are important for short-term endurance:

- High speed and strength levels
- Anaerobic capacity
- Coordination
- High acid tolerance (tolerance of strong muscle hyperacidity)

2   Medium-term endurance (2-10 min)

Medium-term endurance covers individual and team pursuit races on the track in all age groups (2,000-4,000 m) and short road time trials (individual and team). The metabolic rate is still very high but considerably less than that during short-term endurance. The body's oxygen requirement cannot be met during exercise so that part of the energy must be provided anaerobically. The shorter the duration of the maximal effort, the higher the amount of anaerobically supplied energy (around 20%). The training process to develop medium-term and short-term endurance is more complex and sophisticated than that for long-term endurance, as high demands are placed on both the aerobic and anaerobic capacity. In addition, good levels of speed and strength (as in short-term endurance) must also be present.

3   Long-term endurance

This category is further divided into four different forms:

Long-term endurance I (10-35 min)

In long-term endurance I, maximal loading of the cardiovascular system and breathing are still reached. The aerobic capacity (high VO$_2$max) plays a key role. Both heart rate and respiration reach almost maximal levels. Time trials, short school races, and some track races (points races in some categories, knock-out races) fall into the long-term endurance I category. Since about 85% of the energy supply is met aerobically, depleted glycogen stores (muscle glycogen) are a limiting factor. Average lactate levels must be tolerated for relatively long periods (up to 35 min). Fat oxidation does not yet play a key role.

Long-term endurance II (35-90 min)

Loads lasting 35-90 minutes are very common in cycling, as, for example, this includes all races up to a distance of 60 km (e.g., all school, youth, and junior races), as well as all individual time trials (with the exception of junior road races up to 120 km). Muscle and liver glycogen and also fats are used for energy provision, and the aerobic–anaerobic ratio increases to 90:10. A suitably well-developed anaerobic capacity is, however, required for tactical maneuvers like sprint finishes, breakaway attempts, the last miles of a race, or the final spurt.

Long-term endurance III (90 min-6 hr)

Long-term endurance III covers almost all amateur road racing and bike touring, as well as most circuit races and road races. Most professional races do not exceed 6 hours. The energy flow is low compared to the previous categories and allows for a higher proportion of fat burning.

The 90- to 120-minute area, however, still does not have the same characteristics as long-term endurance III and constitutes the transition area between long-term endurance II and III. In general, the transitions between each category are not fixed.

The anerobic threshold is over 90% of VO_2max for very well-trained cyclists, so that even at levels of 3 mmol/l blood a very high pace can still be maintained. Muscle and liver glycogen stores are again performance-limiting, so that it is always necessary to eat carbohydrates during the training or race. Fluids and electrolytes must also be consumed due to the high sweat losses in order to stop your performance from deteriorating.

Long-term endurance IV (over 6 hr)

Exercise durations in excess of 6 hours take place in professional training camps or in extreme cycling tours, where distances of over 250 km (155 mi) are the norm; there are even races, such as the Paris–Bordeaux in France that are longer than 500 km (311 mi). After the muscle and liver glycogen is exhausted, the fat metabolism takes over (80%) aided by gluconeogenesis (i.e., glucose formation from lactate, proteins, and fats). Large quantities of food (carbohydrate) and liquid intake are essential to be able to complete such extreme endurance performances.

In view of the fact that people now compete in triple ultra-triathlons or the Race Across America (RAAM), a long-term endurance V category should now be introduced.

Theoretical principles of strength

The different types of strength are described only briefly here. Sports science has traditionally identified three main types of strength, along with many subforms:

a. Maximal strength
b. Speed strength
c. Strength endurance

Maximal strength refers to the strength an athlete can exert voluntarily during maximum muscular contraction.

Speed strength is the athlete's ability to overcome resistance with fast muscle contraction speed and is highly influenced by the level of *maximum strength*. According to recent studies, maximal strength plays a much more important role than had previously been thought as the foundation of all other types of strength, even for road cycling. *Speed strength* is very important in road cycling, particularly in springs and attacks.

Strength endurance is the ability to withstand fatigue over frequently-repeated strength loads. In mountain sections and breakaway attempts in which gear ratios of up to 53 x 11 are used, *strength endurance* is vital. A simple equation involving strength and cadence states that the higher the cadence at constant speed, the lower the effort; the lower the cadence at constant speed, the greater the effort. Chapter 3.8 explores strength training with and without the bike in greater detail.

Theoretical principles of speed

There are two main types of *speed*: the speed of a single movement (movement speed) and speed of locomotion (riding speed). Movements may either be *cyclical* or *acyclical*. The cycling action is a repetitive (i.e., cyclical movement which is why cyclical speed is of the utmost importance for the cyclist). Cyclical speed (movement speed) is dependent on the gear ratio. For high gear ratios (52 x 12), the cadence and also the movement speed is low. However, the traveling speed can be very high.

Speed can be limited by

- muscle strength,
- reaction speed,
- general aerobic dynamic endurance,
- coordination (inter and intramuscular),
- contraction speed of the muscles, and
- muscle elasticity.

If a high cadence combined with really high effort (high gear ratio, strength endurance) can be maintained for long periods, high traveling speeds can be attained. This shows how dependent speed is on strength; high speeds cannot be achieved without appropriate levels of strength. Both speed and strength should be worked on in training.

Theoretical principles of flexibility

Flexibility is the ability to perform a movement with the largest possible range of motion. Flexibility is more important in sports like gymnastics than in cycling. However, flexibility should not be underestimated as a requirement for peak cycling performance. General flexibility should be improved by means of specific programs and definitely be more developed than in non-athletes.

Flexibility is an essential prerequisite for high-quality movement, and good flexibility helps to prevent injury. In a fall, if the joints and ligaments lack a good range of motion, they can be torn more easily, and even bone fractures are more likely. Inadequate flexibility hinders the development of an athlete's conditioning and coordination. Flexibility increases the movement efficiency of cycling and promotes recovery. Flexibility is very dependent on muscle elasticity, which is why stretching and exercises have a whole chapter devoted to them.

In a direct comparison of two equally strong athletes, the loser will always be the one who is unable to make the most of his other conditioning abilities (endurance, strength, speed, coordination) due to his limited flexibility. The conditioning abilities are interdependent. Too much strength training reduces flexibility and endurance, and it is thought that too much flexibility can negatively impact speed. As in all training, it is up to the individual to find out what works for him.

Theoretical principles of coordination

Coordination is the athlete's ability to exert maximum force with minimal and targeted muscle effort. We differentiate between *intermuscular* and *intramuscular coordination*. Intermuscular coordination is the interaction of muscles, agonist and antagonist; intramuscular coordination concerns the joint action of the central nervous system and a muscle unit (motor unit). The goal of intramuscular training must be to solicit as many muscle units as possible, in order to attain maximal speed in an attack (see chapter 3.8). In cycling, a great deal of cycling-specific coordination is required, while a cyclist's general coordination is usually poorly developed. Co-ordination and flexibility training are often neglected by newcomers to the sport, and this deficit is then never made up. However, cycling-specific coordination may be excellent. Smooth pedaling action, starting off, cornering, and balancing show very highly-developed coordination skills. In order to counteract a loss of general coordination due to the uniform pedaling action from a young age, general coordination should be encouraged (e.g., continued training indoors in the winter). This also has a positive influence on learning new cycling-specific movement forms.

3.2   Training Methodology

Endurance training methodology

There are four different types of endurance training methods, which can be further divided into other methods:

1. The endurance training method is primarily used to build up basic endurance and is divided into:

    a. the continuous method,
    b. the alternating method, and
    c. fartlek.

The continuous method is the main method used in cycling, especially in the preparation phases, as it improves aerobic capacity and recovery ability at low intensities. The exercise duration should be longer than one hour and can last five to eight hours. The training intensity can either remain constant or vary slightly between zones.

a. Continuous method: constant intensity; this is when training load can be most ac-curately controlled by heart rate.

b. Alternating method: the pace is increased to the anaerobic zone over predetermi-ned course sections.

c. Fartlek: the pace is adapted to the terrain and wind conditions.

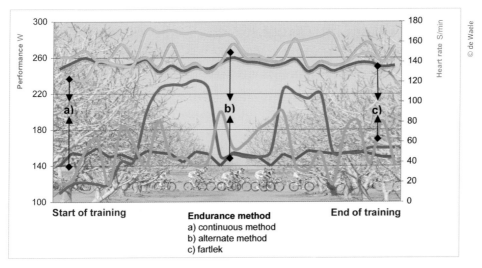

Fig. 3.5: Endurance methods

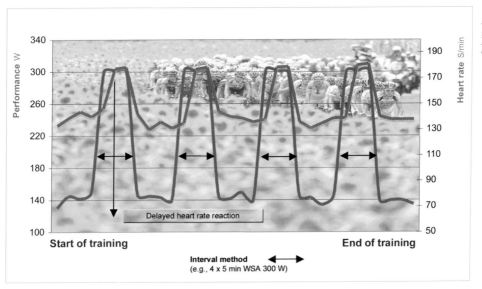

Fig. 3.6: Interval method

2. The interval method involves the systematic alternating of exercise and rest; the rest interval is not long enough to allow for complete recovery, but a new interval is started once the heart rate drops to about 130 bpm. For example, the interval method may be used for sprint training (e.g., 8 x 7 seconds, or 6 x 30 seconds). If several sets are performed, a less common method in cycling, longer rest breaks should be inserted between each set of 4-8 repetitions.

3. The repetition method is characterized by complete recovery rest breaks (heart rate below 100 bpm) between intervals ridden at or above race intensity. This method is not commonly used in cycle racing but is very common in track cycling (e.g., sessions of 3 x 1,000 m).

4. Racing and monitoring methods involve a one-off effort at race intensity and duration. The physiological training load is very similar to that of a typical race in terms of course length and speed and over-distance training (i.e., when the training distance is longer than the race distance), with effort and intensity slightly below race level and slightly above race level in under-distance training. These methods require considerable motivation in order to be able to simulate a race performance. Training races around a circuit are ideal for this, as they simulate the physical, technical, tactical, and mental aspects of actual races. The race method should, however, only be used at the end of the preparation phase or even just at the start of the competition phase. See chapter 3.5 for more information on periodization phases. Time trials (over/under distance; see also chapter 4.3) are used for performance monitoring (monitoring method) and simple performance testing.

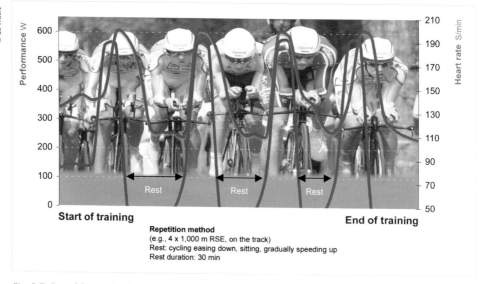

Repetition method
(e.g., 4 x 1,000 m RSE, on the track)
Rest: cycling easing down, sitting, gradually speeding up
Rest duration: 30 min

Fig. 3.7: Repetition method

Strength training methodology

In strength training, training content is described in terms of reps and sets; one set can consist of up to 20 or more reps, performed consecutively without a break although there is a recovery break between the sets.

Speed training methodology

For speed training, see the section on speed training in chapter 3.3.

Flexibility training methodology

Well-developed flexibility is required for a high physical performance level. You should aim for very good cycling-specific and adequate general flexibility. Once you attain optimal flexibility, you must keep it up otherwise you can very quickly revert to the starting level. Choose exercises that are appropriate for the race or training-specific activity, and perform them either during the warm-up or cool-down phases of the workout. More on improving flexibility can be found in chapter 3.9.

Coordination training methodology

Coordination and cycling technique are closely linked, which is why many coordination training tips can be found in the technique section. Coordination training without a bike takes place indoors in winter but should be continued throughout the season.

Coordination training should always be performed when the body is fresh and not at the end of a tough workout when coordination would be reduced. A workout to develop a round pedaling action could, for example, be combined very well with a compensatory recovery session. Cycling technique practice, such as clearing obstacles, touching the rear wheel of the rider in front with your own front wheel, or riding curves can be performed on a rest day (training camp). It is important not to neglect general coordination in your haste to improve your cycling-specific coordination, as it facilitates the learning of new skills on the bike.

3.3   Training Zones

Training is divided into zones to facilitate planning. The zones group exercise according to its intensity and type. This chapter merely presents each zone, while sections 3.5 and 3.6 explain combining and using the training zones and provide example training plans for each category. Studying chapters 2, 3.1, and 3.2 will make it much easier to understand the following.

The heart rates given below relate to an assumed maximal heart rate of 200 bpm. The lactate values are averages for cyclists.

Compensatory training (CT)

Compensatory training helps the body recover from exercise or create a recovery deficit by means of active, sport-specific recovery. CT intensity is the lowest of all training types.

Basic endurance training (BE)

Basic endurance training is definitely the most important type of training for all endurance sports and particularly for cycling. It develops the key performance foundation, a high aerobic capacity, without which a high performance level cannot be attained in cycling. Depending on age, training condition, and discipline, 70-90% of all training mileage is done in the basic endurance zone. Also, a large part of winter training without the racing bike takes place in this zone. Basic endurance training sessions are characterized by large to very large volumes and low intensity. The basic endurance zone is further divided into two intensity levels: basic endurance 1 and basic endurance 2.

Compensatory training (CT)

Description	Recovery training to regain performance ability after intensive training and racing and to warm up before and cool down after exercise.
Heart rate	80-120 bpm
Metabolism	Purely aerobic, lipolysis Lactate acid below 2,0 mmol/l
Volume	15-50 km, flat
Duration	30 min to 2 hrs
Cadence	70-100 rpm
Gear ratio	4.60-6.00 m 42 x 20-16
Methods	Endurance method
Periodization	Used throughout the year, but less so in PP I and II, an important component of microcycles in the ompetition phase
Cyclization	Especially after intensive races and workouts, usually on Mondays and before a race
Organization type	Individual and group training
Tips	Put as little pressure as possible on the pedals, dress warmly; technique can be incorporated into CT training, very important component in training camps when riding out

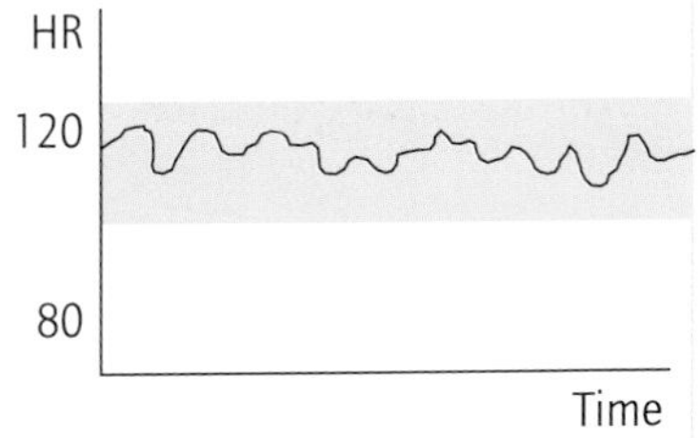

Fig. 3.8: Compensatory training

Basic endurance 1 (BE1)

In workouts lasting between two to over seven hours (with the road bike 60 to over 200 km), the energy supply is exclusively aerobic with a high fat-burning element. This training zone is excellent for fat burning and is the most beneficial from a health point of view (overweight).

Basic endurance 1 (BE1)	
Description	Important training zone for mountain bikers in order to create a high aerobic capacity as the foundation of a high performance level and to warm up before training or racing.
Heart rate	115-145 bpm
Metabolism	Purely aerobic Lactate acid 0-3.0 mmol/l
Volume	50-250 km/31-155 mi, flat to undulating
Duration	2-8 hrs
Cadence	80-110 rpm, opt. 100 rpm
Gear ratio	4.70-6.40 m, z. B. 42 x 19-14
Methods	Duration method
Periodization	Used throughout the year, particularly important in the preparation phase; stick to aerobic zone BE 1 in all other cross-training sports in the PPs; it is an essential element of a spring training camp.
Cyclization	As far as possible train in blocks: 3:1, 4:1, or 5:1 (e.g., 3 hr, 4 hr, 5 hr, 1 hr CT) during the competition phase ideally from Tuesday to Thursday if weekends are race-free, or in the preparation phase from Friday to Sunday.
Organization type	Training alone is the most effective; monitor intensity via heart rate; change leader frequently in group training in order to maintain constant intensity (1-2 min).
Tips	Try to determine individual heart rate values via performance testing, if possible do not train above 150 bpm, a range of about 20 bpm. is optimal, speed is not a monitoring parameter.

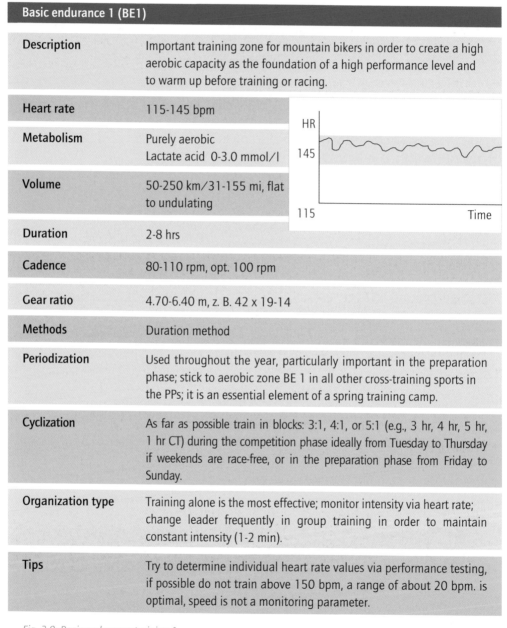

Fig. 3.9: Basic endurance training 1

Basic endurance training 2 (BE2)

The BE2 zone trains the aerobic–anaerobic transition zone. Training can either be strength- or cadence-oriented.

Basic endurance 2 (BE2; strength)	
Description	Medium-intensity training zone to build up race-specific endurance and raise the anaerobic threshold, improve lactate elimination, and optimize the aerobic–anaerobic transition, strength or motor skills training.
Heart rate	About 145-175 bpm
Metabolism	Aerobic–anaerobic transition Aerobic emphasis Lactic acid 3.0-6.0 mmol/l
Volume (road)	5-70 km/3-43.5 mi, flat to undulating
Duration	15 min – 2 hrs
Cadence	70-85 rpm
Gear ratio	6.20-8.60 m (e.g., 52 x 18 – 52 x 13)
Methods	Interval method, repetition method
Periodization	In PP II and III and particularly in the CP, although the longer the race, the less BE 2 training is carried out.
Cyclization	During the CP, advisable on Wednesdays and possibly also Thursdays
Organization type	Training alone: self-motivation not easy, monitor intensity via heart rate and cadence. Group training: frequent change of leader in order to maintain constant intensity (1-2 min).
Tips	Important to establish individual heart rate values using performance testing, range of 10-15 beats is optimal, speed is not a monitoring parameter, use for pre-race warm-up, the volume relates to the whole BE 2 distance covered.

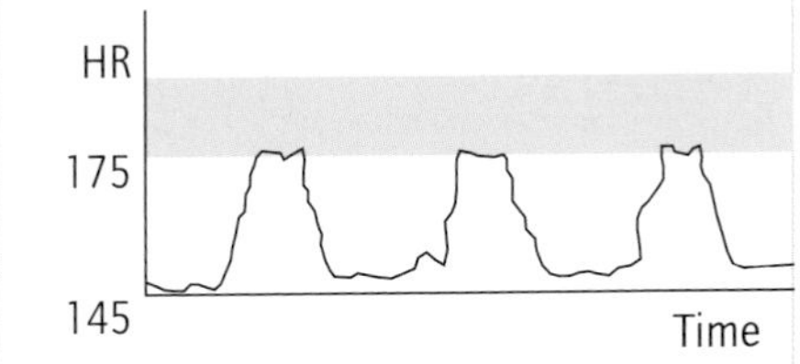

Alongside the Heart rate / Metabolism rows:

HR / 175 / 145 / Time

(e.g., 3 x 8 km) BE 2 interspersed with 15-minute CT sections (HR about 100), Important: warm-up/cool-down

Fig. 3.10: Basic endurance training 2 (strength)

The next section discusses the individual heart rate in the training zones. It is a good idea to add BE 2 intervals to a BE 1 workout.

A long training ride carried out exclusively in the BE 2 zone (over 2-3 hr) is very exhausting and empties the glycogen stores, which is desirable for carbohydrate loading, for example (see chapter 5).

Basic endurance 2 (BE2; cadence)

Description	Medium-intensity training zone to build up race-specific endurance and raise the anaerobic threshold, improve lactate elimination, and optimize the aerobic–anaerobic transition, motor skills training.
Heart rate	About 145-175 bpm
Metabolism	Aerobic–anaerobic transition Lactate acid 3.0-5.0 mmol/l
Volume	5-70 km/3-43.5 mi, flat to undulating
Duration	15 min – 2 hrs
Cadence	100-120 rpm
Gear ratio	5.60-7.60 m (e.g,. 42 x 16-52 x 15)
Methods	Interval method, repetition method
Periodization	In PP III and the CP, and particularly in race preparation, the longer the race, the less BE 2 training is necessary.
Cyclization	During the CP, on Wednesdays and also Thursdays advisable as well as a short BE 2 course the day before a race
Organization type	Training alone: self-motivation not easy, monitor intensity via heart rate and cadence. Group training: frequent change of leader in order to maintain constant intensity (1-2 min).
Tips	Important to establish individual heart rate values using performance testing, range of 10-15 beats is optimal, speed is not a monitoring parameter, use for pre-race warm-up, the volume relates to the whole BE 2 distance covered.

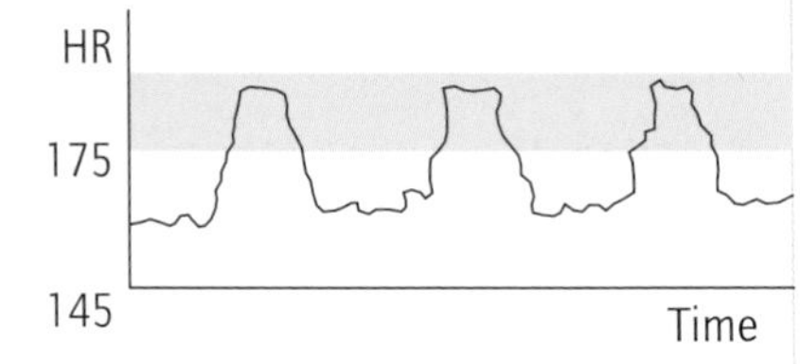

(e.g. 3 x 8 km) BE 2 interspersed with min CT sections (HR approx. 100) Important: warm-up/cool-down

Fig. 3.11: Basic endurance training 2 (cadence)

Race-specific endurance (RSE)

Training in the RSE zone is focused, as the name suggests, on racing speed and effort. Depending on fitness, sections are ridden at racing intensity or higher. Training in the race-specific zone can be performed with very high cadence and low power, with racing cadences and racing gear ratios, or with high gear ratios and correspondingly low cadences and high power. In group training, the leaders should not stay at the front for longer than 60 seconds in order to guarantee an even load for each cyclist. Another form of RSE training is motor-paced training, carried out in the wind shadow of a motorbike or car, which improves both speed endurance and motor skills.

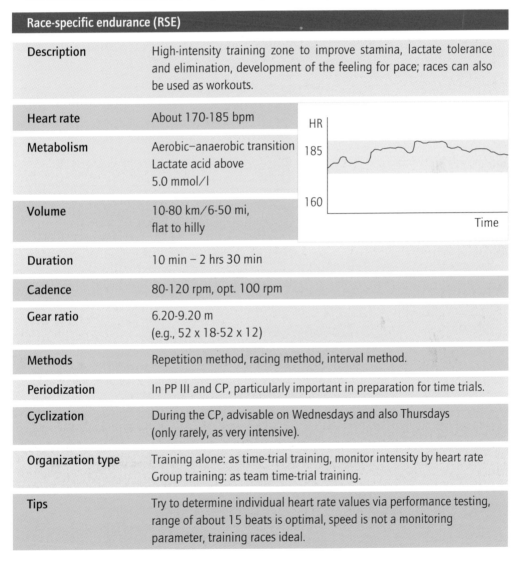

Race-specific endurance (RSE)	
Description	High-intensity training zone to improve stamina, lactate tolerance and elimination, development of the feeling for pace; races can also be used as workouts.
Heart rate	About 170-185 bpm
Metabolism	Aerobic–anaerobic transition Lactate acid above 5.0 mmol/l
Volume	10-80 km/6-50 mi, flat to hilly
Duration	10 min – 2 hrs 30 min
Cadence	80-120 rpm, opt. 100 rpm
Gear ratio	6.20-9.20 m (e.g., 52 x 18-52 x 12)
Methods	Repetition method, racing method, interval method.
Periodization	In PP III and CP, particularly important in preparation for time trials.
Cyclization	During the CP, advisable on Wednesdays and also Thursdays (only rarely, as very intensive).
Organization type	Training alone: as time-trial training, monitor intensity by heart rate Group training: as team time-trial training.
Tips	Try to determine individual heart rate values via performance testing, range of about 15 beats is optimal, speed is not a monitoring parameter, training races ideal.

Fig. 3.12: Race-specific endurance

Special training zones
The special training zones account for a very small percentage of total training.

Speed training (ST)
Speed training is one of the special training zones and is not the same as speed strength training. Speed here does not mean cycling speed but movement speed, which in cycling terms means cadence. Both pure speed and speed endurance are trained.

Speed training (ST)	
Description	High-intensity training zone above the anaerobic threshold to improve speed and speed endurance as well as lactate tolerance and stamina.
Heart rate	Above anaerobic threshold > 175 bpm
Metabolism	Anaerobic Lactate acid above 6.0 mmol/l
Volume	0.5-5 km/0.3-3 mi, flat
Duration	40 sec – 8 min
Cadence	120 – max. rpm
Gear ratio	5.20–7.50 m, (e.g., 42 x 17 – 52 x 15)
Methods	Interval method
Periodization	In PP II and III at the end of each phase and in the CP, particularly important in the preperation for track races and criteriums.
Cyclization	During the CP, on Tuesdays and also advisable on Wednesdays (only rarely, as very intensive).
Organization type	Individual training: intensity monitoring by cadence. Group training: improves motivation, easier to maintain high cadence.
Tips	Wise to establish individual heart rates via performance testing; speed is not a monitoring parameter, perform regularly; performance monitoring: maximum cadence test.

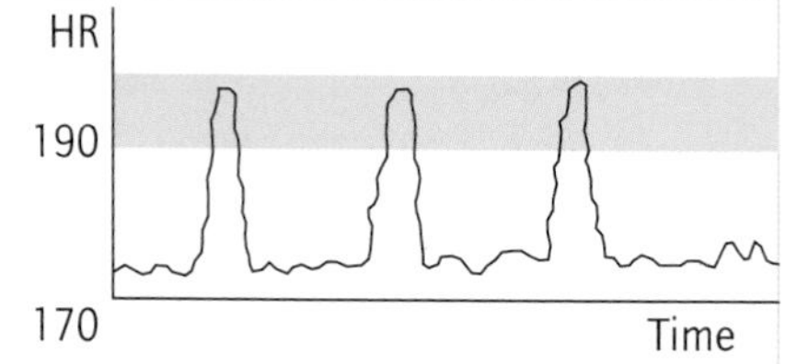

(e.g., 3 x 1000 m) ST interspersed with CT/BE 1 sections gear ratio (e.g., 42 x 16 or 3 x 1 min) Important: warm up/cool-down

Fig. 3.13: Speed training

Speed strength or sprint training (SS)

Speed strength training serves to improve sprinting and acceleration ability. The training forms are covered in detail in chapter 3.8.

With medium gear ratios, start from a very slow speed or a stationary position, then accelerate as fast as possible for 6-8 seconds and then ride on slowly, then repeat after 1-3 minutes.

SS training is particularly important for circuit and track cyclists.

Speed strength training (SS)	
Description	Specific, high-intensity training zone to improve speed and maximum strength; improvement of the anaerobic–alactic metabolism.
Heart rate	Not relevant
Metabolism	Anaerobic-alactic, Lactate ⇔ 2.5 (4.0) mmol/l
Volume	Include 60 km BE 1session
Duration	6-12 x 6 sec, 1-3 sets
Cadence	Maximum from a standing position
Gear ratio	6.2-7.2 m, (e.g., 52 x 18 – 52 x 15)
Methods	Interval method, rest length 3-5 min
Periodization	In PP II and III and in the CP, particularly important in the preparation of track races, circuit races, and criteriums.
Cyclization	Recommended during CP on Tuesdays and also Wednesdays.
Organization type	Training alone: monitor intensity by timing (6-8 sec) Group training: increases motivation, makes it easier to keep going during the reps.
Tips	Maximum pedaling but for only 6, at most 8 sec, but at 100% effort; start off with easy gears, speed is not a monitoring parameter; perform regularly.

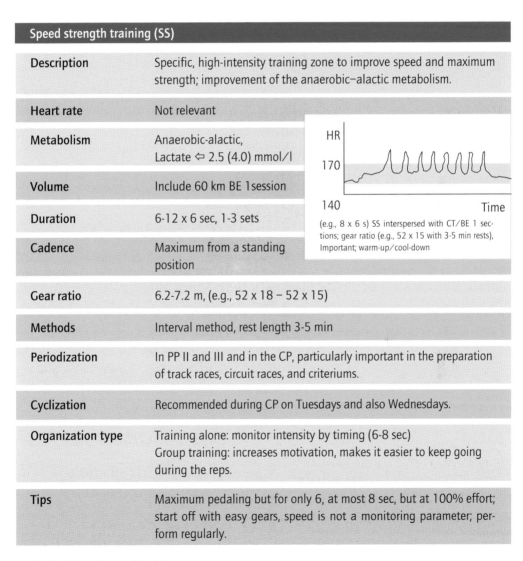

(e.g., 8 x 6 s) SS interspersed with CT/BE 1 sections; gear ratio (e.g., 52 x 15 with 3-5 min rests), Important; warm-up/cool-down

Fig. 3.14: Speed strength training

Strength endurance training (SE)

The aim of strength endurance training is to improve the ability to withstand fatigue when performing high, cyclically-repeating strength loads. In order to be able to train with increased resistance, the training rides should be performed on a mountain or pass with a gentle incline. With a high gear ratio (large wheel), the relatively flat incline is tackled with a cadence of

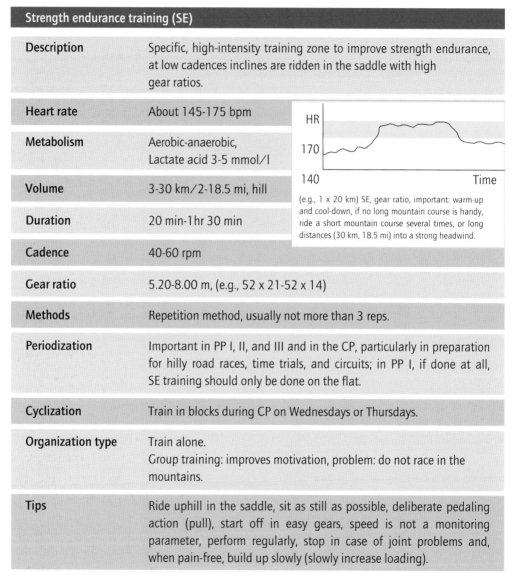

Strength endurance training (SE)	
Description	Specific, high-intensity training zone to improve strength endurance, at low cadences inclines are ridden in the saddle with high gear ratios.
Heart rate	About 145-175 bpm
Metabolism	Aerobic-anaerobic, Lactate acid 3-5 mmol/l
Volume	3-30 km/2-18.5 mi, hill
Duration	20 min-1hr 30 min
Cadence	40-60 rpm
Gear ratio	5.20-8.00 m, (e.g., 52 x 21-52 x 14)
Methods	Repetition method, usually not more than 3 reps.
Periodization	Important in PP I, II, and III and in the CP, particularly in preparation for hilly road races, time trials, and circuits; in PP I, if done at all, SE training should only be done on the flat.
Cyclization	Train in blocks during CP on Wednesdays or Thursdays.
Organization type	Train alone. Group training: improves motivation, problem: do not race in the mountains.
Tips	Ride uphill in the saddle, sit as still as possible, deliberate pedaling action (pull), start off in easy gears, speed is not a monitoring parameter, perform regularly, stop in case of joint problems and, when pain-free, build up slowly (slowly increase loading).

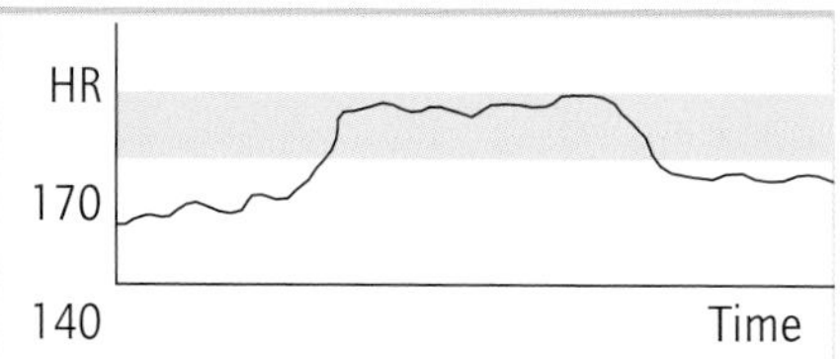
HR
170
140
Time

(e.g., 1 x 20 km) SE, gear ratio, important: warm-up and cool-down, if no long mountain course is handy, ride a short mountain course several times, or long distances (30 km, 18.5 mi) into a strong headwind.

Fig. 3.15: Strength endurance training

between 40 and 60 per minute in the sitting position. This is an excellent way of working on the smooth pedaling action, particularly the pull phase. When training on flat terrain, it is best to carry out SE training with maximum gear ratios against a headwind in order to achieve a similar training effect.

If the heart rate reaches maximum levels, it means that the strength load is too low and the cadence too high, and a higher gear ratio must be used.

A good way of developing race-specific strength endurance is to ride a mountain course of at least 4-km long with racing gear ratios, including simulations of several (3-5) breakaway attempts over 300 m, in which the gear ratio is increased. End with a finishing sprint over the last 500 m. This method should only be used very rarely as it is very intensive.

If you do not have access to mountains on which to perform SE training, a flat course can also be used. If possible on a flat course, ride into a strong, constant headwind, although this only produces the same results with the highest gear ratios.

Strength training has gained importance in recent years, for higher and higher speeds are targeted, especially with greater gear ratios. The high strength load and low movement frequency ensure that the intensity remains in the submaximal zone.

Because of the high strength load, this method can cause blood pressure spikes, making it inappropriate for therapeutic cyclists. You can read more about the application of each training zone in chapters 3.5 and 3.6.

3.4   Using a Heart Rate Monitor

This chapter is intended to show the different ways of using heart rate monitors and how they work. Tips are also given on how to determine the training zones. Finally, the most common training errors are covered.

How does a heart rate monitor work?

As little as 20 years ago, monitoring heart rate training was a gamble, as the pulse could only be measured at certain points of the body (wrist, neck), which made continuous heart rate measurement impossible. People also lacked experience when it came to interpreting the heart rate data. The first heart rate monitors were only used by top athletes, who were able to achieve great success using this method. The unbelievable success of the East German cyclists was based, among other things, on the consistent development and application of heart rate-orien-

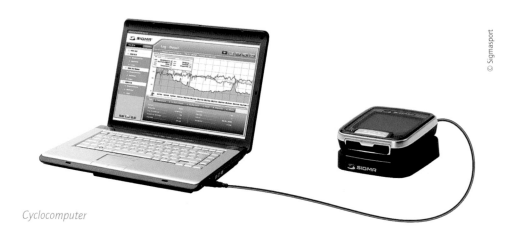

© Sigmasport

Cyclocomputer

ted training. Already in the mid-70s the first trials were being made with wireless hear rate mo-nitors. In the mid-80s, the first completely functional heart rate monitors by Polar hit the mar-ket, and today the heart rate monitor is an essential training monitoring tool available to all (around $30). Heart rate monitors are now used by everyone from elite amateurs or pros to hobby cyclists.

The heart rate is picked up by a transmitter integrated in a chest strap and transmitted wire-lessly by radio to the watch (receiver). The heart beat is captured by the chest electrodes loca-ted in the strap according to the ECG method. All other methods, such as taking the pulse with the fingers, are considerably less accurate.

User-friendly models allow for programming the desired training intensity zone and give an acoustic or visual signal if you exceed or drop below it. The top of the range models by Polar allow you to store heart rate data and other performance parameters (speed, cadence) during training or racing. At home, these data can then be transferred to a computer, where they can be shown in graph form and analyzed. The data provide important information for effective training management.

Moisten your belt!
It is better to put the watch on the handle bar near the stem for better control. When using a heart rate monitor, it is important to position the strap correctly and not too tightly so as not to hinder breathing. The electrodes can only capture the heart rate if they are slightly damp. Either moisten them with a little water prior to training, or ride for a few minutes until contact is obtained thanks to your natural sweat production. In the immediate vicinity of strong power sources (e.g., high voltage cables, railway lines), the monitor may briefly register very high fi-gures or stop altogether.

Occasionally when training in pairs or in a group, there can be interference and disturbance of individual transmitters and receivers, but this is prevented in newer models by coding the transmission frequency that prevents interference between monitors in a cycling group.

Heart rate behavior in cycling

Already when cycling on the flat, the heart rate fluctuates considerably, depending on the course profile, the weather, and the road surface. Normally, cyclists use speed to measure their training intensity, although this is unreliable due to the previously mentioned factors, which is obvious when you consider how much the intensity increases when cycling into a strong head-wind and how much it decreases with a following wind. Thus you need to find an alternative to speed for measuring training intensity.

In modern training science and goal-oriented training, intensity is controlled by heart rate and not by speed, which even on flat terrain is not an indicator of intensity. The desired intensity can be found by adjusting gear ratio and cadence.

One consequence of heart rate-oriented training is that now you must ride more slowly into a headwind or downhill in order to not exceed the desired intensity zone (e.g., BE 1). Of course, the heart rate zones are not set in stone; when circumstances require, it is quite possible to deviate slightly, although the majority of training should take place as planned in the desired zones (usually BE 1).

Resting heart rate (RHR)

As already mentioned in chapter 2.2, the heart rate behavior changes during the training process. In particular, a lower resting heart rate is considered to be an indication of improved endurance ability. Measuring your resting heart rate is a good way of familiarizing yourself with using a heart rate monitor. The RHR is not just a good indicator of endurance fitness, it also warns you about oncoming illnesses, infections, and overtraining. Only by regularly taking your RHR before getting out of bed in the morning can changes be spotted. If your RHR normally lies between 45 and 48 bpm, and then one morning you measure it at 55, this could be an indication that you are coming down with an illness, even if there are no discernable symptoms. If the RHR slowly rises over a period of days, this usually means that you are over-training, or in any case that your recovery is disturbed. After tough races or stage races, the RHR is often raised due to the extreme effort and short recovery times. Generally in the case of an upward deviation of 6-8 bpm, the previous factors should be investigated, and you should train and race cautiously, particularly if the exercise heart rate is also raised. It may even be necessary to halt training prematurely, as endurance training when you are carrying an infection can damage the heart muscle and other organs.

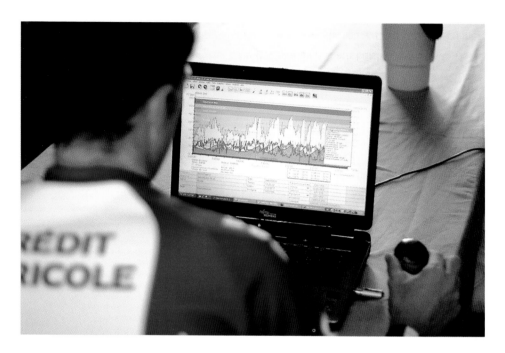

Take your pulse every morning

Measuring your pulse in the morning and entering the result in your training diary should be part of every cyclist's daily routine (chapter 3.10), so that particularly as a cycling newbie, you can trace the evolution of your RHR over months and years. At high performance level, the RHR can be related to other parameters such as race results and represented in graph form. If you don't want to put on your heart rate monitor in the morning, you can also take your pulse manually on the carotid artery, directly on the heart, or on your wrist. You should measure it for 15 seconds and multiply the result by 4. Leaving a pencil and a piece of paper by your bed is a good way to remind yourself to take your pulse before getting up. The approximate values are provided in chapter 2.2. The RHR of children and adolescents is usually around 10 bpm higher than that of adults. Rarely, cyclists with many years of training under their belts may have a constant RHR or up to 80bpm. This is nothing to worry about, as there are always physiological exceptions to the rule, but a medical check is advisable.

Establishing training zones

Most of the training zones described in the previous chapter use the heart rate for monitoring purposes. The values shown correspond to an 18- to 35-year-old cyclist in good physical shape with a maximum pulse rate of about 200 bpm. Younger and older cyclists, and also athletes with varying maximum heart rates, should not use these figures, because they would not be training in the correct zone. That is why each training zone should be established by performance testing or by using the maximum heart rate. The procedure for calculating the training zones using the MHR and the RHR is explained next.

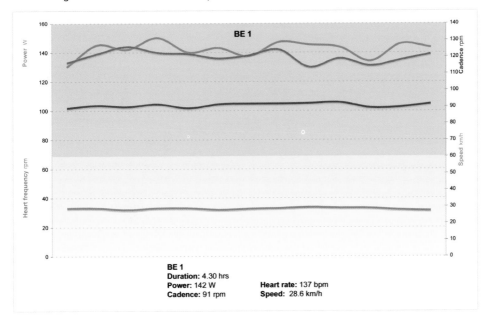

Fig. 3.16: Basic endurance training 1

Determining maximum heart rate (MHR)

The most accurate and safest way to determine MHR is to measure the MHR during a performance test under medical supervision. More senior cyclists (over the age of 40) and beginners should not carry out this test alone but only under medical supervision due to the risks involved. Measuring the MHR would be too risky for rehabilitation cyclists, who may calculate their MHR according to the formula 220 − age = MHR, or using accurate medical testing. Women should use a starting value of 225. However, this formula only gives a very rough approximation (+/-) and should never be used by high-performance cyclists.

Performing the test

After a 30-minute warm-up, start the test to determine MHR. While the test in the summer can be carried out on the bike, in winter it can also be done as a running test, although running and cycling MHRs do differ slightly. In order to reach MHR, the effort should be increasing over a period of several minutes (about 4-5 min), with the last minute ridden flat out.

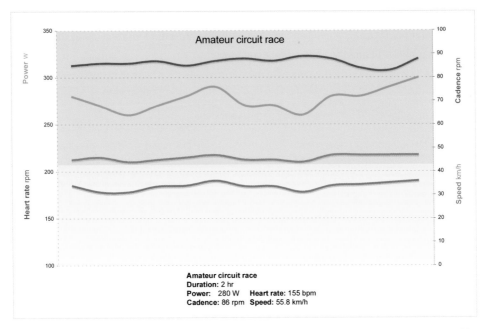

Fig. 3.17: Heart rate behavior during a circuit race (amateur). The leader with a MHR of about 200 rides for almost the entire race at the limit of his endurance ability.

A mountain with a very slight incline of 3-4 km is ideal and should be tackled at racing speed and with racing gear ratios. Over the last 600 m, pick up the pace so that you are riding absolutely flat-out. A high movement frequency (cadence) is necessary to reach your MHR. Right at the end of the test or just afterward, the heart rate is usually at its highest. This test should be carried out on different days in order to minimize any extenuating circumstances.

In most cases, the MHR will lie in the region of 220 – age; exceptions are not impossible though, as trained cyclists often have a maximal heart rate of around 200 until the age of 35 or even older.

The **running test** should ideally be carried out on a 1-2 km (0.6-1.2 mi) flat or slightly inclined course. As in the cycling test, the last 400 m (44 yds) are run at maximum intensity, and the MHR is measured when exhaustion forces you to stop the test. The measurement is only sufficiently accurate with a heart rate monitor and only this result should be used in further calculations. Due to the state of extreme exhaustion at the end of the test, it is impossible to take your pulse manually in any case.

Calculating intensity zones

The formulae used to calculate intensity zones are the product of many years of comprehensive studies of endurance athletes and are therefore very accurate. Determining the training zones with this simple method is a reliable alternative to expensive and complex performance testing. However, performance testing is, of course, more accurate and is mainly used at elite level. But even good amateurs can safely use the method presented here.

The exercise heart rate for each training zone is calculated using the resting heart rate and the maximum heart rate as follows:

1. Subtract the **resting heart rate** from the MHR.

2. Multiply this figure by the **intensity factor**.

3. The **resting heart rate** is added to the result.

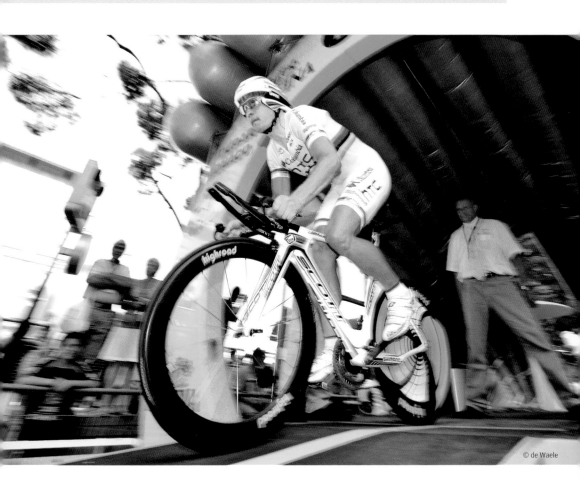

© de Waele

Example:

1.   200 – 45 = 155

2.   155 x 0.52 = 80.6

3.   80.6 + 45 = 125.6

The calculated figure would be the upper heart rate limit for compensatory training (recovery training) for the person concerned. The factors for each intensity zone are listed below:

Table 3.1: Intensity factors

Training zone		Factor
• Compensatory zone	CT	up to 0.52
• Basic endurance 1	BE 1	0.52 – 0.65
• Basic endurance 2	BE 2	0.65 – 0.77
• Race-specific endurance	RSE	0.75 – 0.95
• Strength endurance	SE	0.75 – 0.90
• Speed training	ST	0.85 – 1.00
• Speed strength training	SS	0.85 – 0.95

The factors represent the lower and upper limits of each zone. Correct intensity management is particularly important in the compensatory zone and the basic endurance zones. It doesn't depend on one or two beats and much less on the calculated place after the decimal point. The calculations provide a reference value that can be used as a guide in training.

In the last three specific high-intensity training zones (SE, ST, and SS), training is managed less according to heart rate and more according to specific gear ratio data, cadences, and movement tasks for predetermined time or distance intervals, as a heart rate of 180 bpm, for example, can be attained by different training methods and workloads. However, even in these cases, the correct level of exertion is usually not reflected in the heart rate.

The worst training errors

These are the most important training errors:

- Training is too intensive, mainly in BE 2 and in RSE. The emphasis should be on the development of a high aerobic capacity by means of BE 1. Over-intensive training during the week may prevent peak performance at the weekend. Poor recovery (constant exhaustion) and empty glycogen reserves are symptoms of this state.
- This can often be due to insufficient training in the BE 1 zone.
- Lack of periodization; cyclists have almost the same form throughout the year. No cyclization within the training week.
- Ignoring the laws of recovery.
- Excessive increases in workload and abrupt jumps in the yearly build-up lead to performance stagnation or even deterioration.
- Not cutting down on training in the case of illness or infection often leads to a loss of performance.
- Strength and strength endurance training are completely neglected.
- Monotonous training is often performance-limiting.
- Ignoring new training science discoveries.

Other training errors can be found in the following chapters.

3.5   Training Periodization

What does periodization mean?
Periodization is the division of the training year into periods or phases with different objectives, with an end goal of peaking for a main race. Periodization gives structure to training. It is impossible to compete at the highest level on an ongoing basis, as the body needs time to rest and recover. Over a period of years, the training load should gradually be increased in order to develop the cyclist's potential. This is mainly reflected in an increase in training mileage. This also explains why newcomers to the sport rarely experience success in the first year despite high training mileages.

These criteria apply only partially for recreational cyclists, as they ride their bike when they have the time and inclination, but a simplified periodization is also helpful for them. The classic three-phase periodization looks like this:

1. Preparation phase (PP)

2. Competition phase (CP)

3. Transition phase (TP)

Phases during the year

The *preparation phase* is characterized by foundation training in all areas of conditioning, with special emphasis on endurance as a foundation on which to build in the competition phase.

In the *competition phase*, all training is geared to racing and is therefore more intensive and more structured, normally around a single peak (e.g., national championships). The amount of important races in the calendar makes choosing just one a difficult task. At a high performance level, for Olympic contenders or World Championships participants for example, preparation is clearly focused on a single race. Peak form, which can usually only be maintained for a few weeks or even a few days, must be attained for the race.

This kind of periodization with just one single peak is called *single periodization*. Periodization with two peaks is *double periodization* and with several: *multiple periodization*. The problem with multiple periodization is that absolute peak performances cannot ever be achieved, as the period over which peak form must be maintained is too long. However, multiple periodization is useful for cyclists, particularly for circuit specialists, as this gives them the opportunity to race every weekend and therefore to consider several races in the spring, summer, and early fall as their peaks.

A very good example of double periodization is the elite cyclist who needs to be in peak form in May for qualification races and then needs to peak again in the summer at national and international championships. Double periodization with two competition phases—one on the road in the summer and one on the track or cross-country in the winter—is extremely rare at elite level, as this requires two completely separate preparation phases which overlap with the preceding competition phases. In the 1960s and 70s, though, it was possible to be world class both at cross-country and on the road.

As the competition phase comes to an end, it leads directly into the transition phase, which involves active recovery and also provides an opportunity to have a mental break from the sport.

Before presenting the training for the different age groups, the different phases should be characterized in more detail, as the fundamental principles are the same for all age groups. I have used the example of a single periodization with one competition phase.

Breakdown of the season

Year-round training is essential when it comes to training planning, as regular training is the only way to improve performance, and a winter break from October to March is no longer possible even for hobby cyclists.

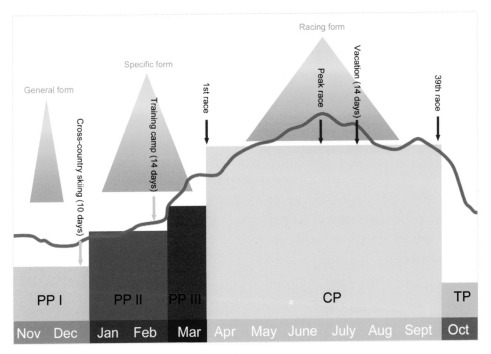

Fig. 3.18: Periodization diagram for road-cycle racing

Preparation phase

This starts around the middle of November and last until the start of the racing season around the middle or end of March, so the phase lasts around five months. As previously mentioned, this is when the foundation for the racing phase is laid. The biggest problem in the whole preparation phase in fall and winter is the short days and poor weather. For this reason, many

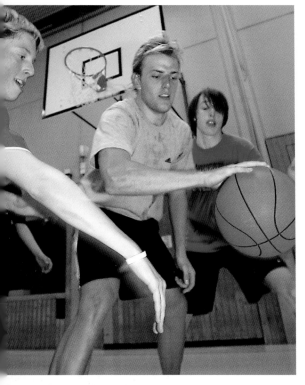
Indoor training

cyclists are only able to train at the weekends on the bike and are forced to exercise indoors in the gym. Running or jogging are good alternatives, although the first running sessions are hard for cyclists (i.e., muscle soreness). It is still possible to run after dark and when it's raining to keep fit during the week with 30- to 60-minute runs. The preparation phase is divided into more sections known as macrocycles, which also have their own goals.

The **first macrocycle** (first preparation phase) from early- to mid-November to the end of December involves a variety of sporting activity that is not restricted to cycling alone. Other endurance sports make a welcome change to the cycling training that has become monotonous toward the end of the season. Sports such as running, swimming, mountain biking, skiing, roller skiing, inline skating, and ice speed skating are all suitable. A well-structured indoor training session led by an experienced coach will improve coordination, strength, speed, flexibility, and also endurance. After a long cycling season, the supporting skeletal muscles need a sensible program of non-sport-specific and build-up training in order to avoid or compensate for postural defects.

Roller skiing is an excellent form of endurance and whole-body training for cyclists in the winter. It can still be practiced regularly even when there is no snow. In very cold weather, it is more pleasant than cycling on the roads (lower speed). The expense of buying a pair of roller skis is always worth it, and the technique can be mastered after just a few training sessions.

Skating and nordic skating

Inline skating is better at targeting cycling-specific muscles. It is not for nothing that Dutch cyclists train on ice speed skating tracks in the winter and ice speed skaters train on bikes in the summer. The multi Olympic medal winning speed skater Eric Heiden also contested the Tour de France, and in women's sport there are several examples of medal winners both on the bike and on blades. In the absence of a suitable ice speed skating track, inline skating is a good alternative, as it perfectly simulates the speed skating action. On quiet roads and cycle paths, this will enable you to cover distances of 10-40 km (6-25 mi) in the basic endurance zones. If you add a couple of cross-country ski poles with asphalt rubber tips, you can train your whole body with Nordic skating.

For all activities in the preparation phase, the emphasis should be on fun and variety. The intensity is almost exclusively in the BE 1 and BE 2 zones, with emphasis on BE 1 training. Of course, some training, especially in the gym and on the mountain bike, will exceed these zones and also trigger certain adaptation processes. It is a good idea to use a mountain bike for road training in cold weather. Due to the higher rolling friction, lower speeds are achieved with the same effort, which is beneficial in cold weather as then the body cools down less quickly. **Mountain biking** off-road noticeably improves bike handling and cycling technique. Nevertheless, training should be carried out on the racing bike at least once a week.

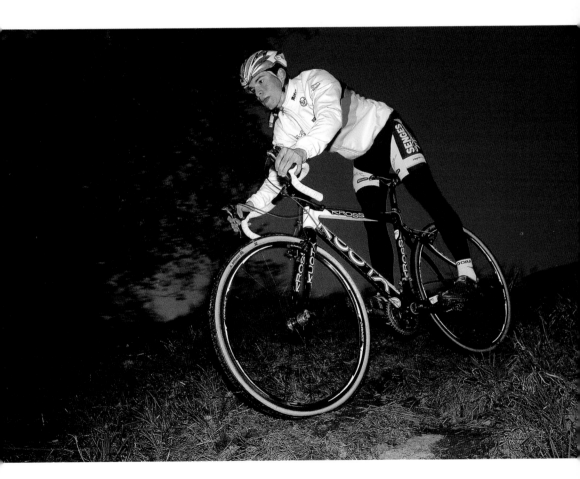

The weekend is the perfect time for training on the bike. Regularity is also important in this section of the training year; there should be as few days or even weeks of training lost as possible (except in the case of illness). Training sessions in winter are considerably shorter than in the summer and last between one and three, sometimes four, hours. Toward the end of the first macrocycle, the training volume increases significantly.

Second macrocycle

The **second macrocycle** (second preparation phase) runs from the beginning of January until the end of February. It starts with a recovery week in which training is very light. Without reducing the other training methods, specific training, such as bike training in the BE 1 zone, increases in the second macrocycle. Not until February does bike training gradually squeeze out the other sports, though one or two should still occasionally be practiced as non-cycling specific activities during the season.

A macrocycle is divided into several **microcycles**, which is just another name for weekly training plans. The volume and intensity of each micro- and macrocycle should not remain constant, which makes their structure particularly important. Ratios of training to rest of 2:1, 3:1, 4:1, or even 5:1 are usual. The first number indicates the number of weeks with increasing training load, and the second number indicates a following week with light training for recovery. The same ratio is also used for daily workouts (microcycles), where training load increases over two to five days followed by a compensatory day. Specific training (strength endurance, speed, and speed strength training) are often carried out both during the preparation phases and during the season in blocks of two to four days with increasing training load (e.g., 1st day: 3 km SE, 2nd day: 8 km SE, 3rd day: 2 x 8 km SE). In the course of the second macrocycle, training volume and frequency are increased, while intensity still remains in the basic endurance zones. Then there is another week of light training or a few days of reduced training for recovery purposes. Whether you train for two or five days or weekly blocks depends on your fitness levels. Blocks with the ratio 3:1 have been used successfully by all age groups.

The **third macrocycle** (third preparation phase) starts at the beginning of March and lasts right up until racing starts or even after the first preparation races. After this cycle you should be in racing form or should be able to achieve racing form after the first racing phase, depending on your objective. A top amateur must already be at peak fitness at the end of March and beginning of April for the first classics, while lower-ranked amateurs or cyclists of other age groups who are under less pressure to succeed will be able to take things more slowly. This is particularly the case for hobby cyclists. Elite cyclists must ride more and increase intensity sooner. The cycle described here is classic periodization based on the racing season. Such a long season may not be a great idea, as it is also possible to consider periodizations that are shifted so that the racing phase does not start until May or June and continues with no downtime right to the end of the season. The advantages of this are obvious; first the phase with highest training volume is shifted to a warmer time of year and then peak form is reached when many other cyclists are already feeling jaded. In September and the beginning of October, good performances can still be achieved. This periodization is recommended for young cyclists and newcomers to the sport. However, this should just make you think about the various other variations.

Back to the classic model: If possible, a two-week training camp should be planned at the beginning of March (see chapter 3.7), although this can also take place later in the year. The final two to three weeks before the season starts are used to train specific abilities like strength, speed, and race-specific endurance. To this end, training intensities, as previously mentioned, are increased and varied according to objectives from the start of the third macrocycle.

Racing phase

The racing season can stretch from mid-March to mid-October, a long time to maintain your performance level. The division of the racing phase depends on the cyclist's goals. If you need to peak during a certain period, the individual training plan can be structured around this. For example, if you need to peak at the beginning of June, the direct preparation starts in April. In two phases lasting three to four weeks, training increases for two or three weeks, and for a few days at the end of each phase, training is significantly reduced particularly on the days just before races. The second phase starts with a load that corresponds to the average load in the first phase, and the load increases significantly to the value of the highest load of the first phase. In the first week before the race, training is mostly geared to recovery, and this is also the time in which carbohydrate loading may be carried out (see chapter 5.3).

The choice of races or bike tours should also range from easy to harder (e.g., longer, more hilly) in order to manage performance development. Ideally, include multiday circuit races in the third week or both phases. After the peak at the beginning of June, form is usually maintained for one to two weeks. After this, training is slightly lighter so that the form gradually drops. At the start of July, the process can be repeated in order to be able to peak again in September and October.

Cyclization

In the racing phase, microcycle structure is critically important.

Monday

Mondays are usually recovery days involving compensatory training. Many racing cyclists either do not train on Mondays or practice a different sport.

Tuesday

Tuesdays are for sprint or strength training combined with a short- to medium-length BE 1 session. If you are still too tired after racing at the weekend, just do the BE 1 training.

Wednesday

On Wednesdays, carry out a ride that is longer than the one on Tuesday at BE 1 or BE 2 intensity. Intervals in the RSE zone can also be performed (e.g., 3 x 5 km with 52 x 15, complete recovery).

Thursday

On Thursdays, carry out a long BE 1 session that is significantly longer than the race distance (overdistance). Youth cyclists can cover distances of up to 120 km, juniors up to 180 km, and amateurs up to more than 220 km. These distances are the farthest and should not be ridden regularly by U-19 age groups, for a weekly training distance of 180 km would for average junior cyclists be excessive. On vacation, when cyclists have enough time, such long rides can be included over several weeks.

Friday

On the Fridays before Saturday races, go for a really short ride in the CT zone. A few sprints or tempo rides will let you know if you are fit enough and will prepare the body for the following day's race. If you are not racing until Sunday, train on Friday in the BE 1 zone with a few below maximal tempo intervals.

Weekend

Saturdays are for CT training and Sunday is race day. A race-free weekend should be used for one or two long endurance rides that cannot be done during the week due to lack of time.

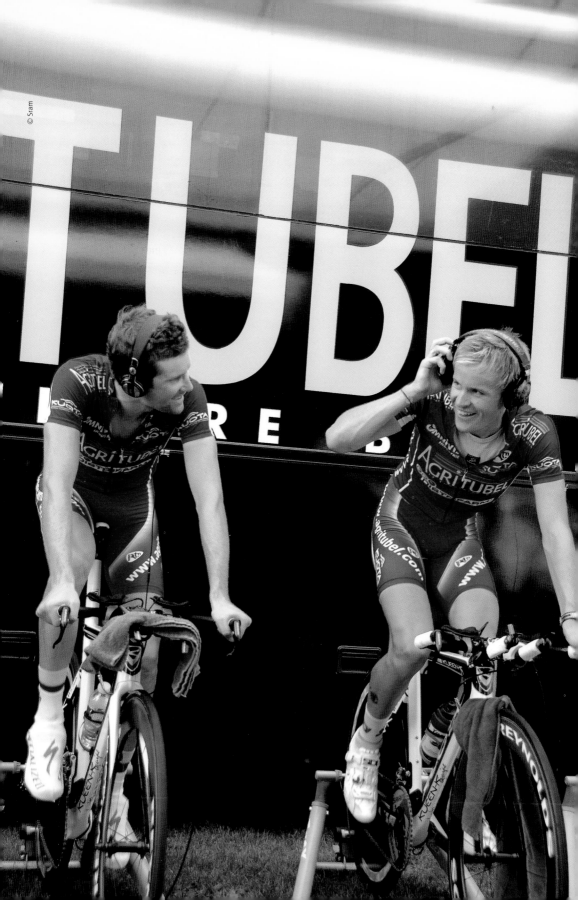

At the start of the racing season in April and May, many amateurs and professionals (in this case in March) add on an extra BE training ride to the race; they cycle home or even to the race for another one to two hours (BE 1). This training method can also be used in other periods of the racing phase for the purposes of performance improvement. However, beware of overtraining after very tough races, as in these cases the additional training would have a detrimental effect.

Transition phase

In October, the racing phase gives way to the transition phase. In the final weeks of the racing phase, the training volume is already dropping The training volume is further reduced in the transition phase, and the specific cycling training almost disappears. In this phase lasting from October to mid-November (sometimes even longer), the cyclist must deliberately shun his bike and practice other sports that he enjoys. If a cross-country or winter track season is scheduled after this, the transition phase is considerably shorter or eliminated completely. In this case, it would be wise to end the road season early (in August or September), have a few days' rest, and then begin a shortened specific preparation cycle. The transition phase will rekindle your enjoyment of cycling and enable you to start preparations for the new season with enthusiasm. Particularly for youth riders, this break from the bike is very important as it allows them to pursue other interests and hobbies. Variety is paramount in this phase and should never be sacrificed in favor of training in the obstinate pursuit of success.

Be your own coach

"Be your own coach" is an American phrase typical of the American approach to sport, particularly endurance sport. You are in the best position to know your body, feel the exhaustion and the strength and are therefore best placed to decide what is right for you in terms of training. However, a certain amount of knowledge is still required for this, which this book attempts to provide. A sensible, self-constructed training plan based on a few important training rules guarantees good performance development. It is up to you to determine a sensible proportion of flexibility and highly structured training in order to be successful while also having fun. Stubbornly and unthinkingly sticking 100% to a rigid program cannot achieve this. Listen to your body and decide what works for you and what doesn't. If you don't feel good after training or racing, rest for a day. Coaches and parents of young cyclists will also find useful tips and ideas in the following section, along with a few comments which may aid training planning.

3.6   Training for Different Categories

This chapter deals more specifically with training for cycling tourists and hobby cyclists as well as the various race categories. One section is also devoted to the health-conscious cyclist who exercises for preventive reasons. For every group, two example weekly training plans are provided for illustrative purposes, one from the preparation phase and one from the season as well as an annual plan. However, one problem must be pointed out here: These training plans are kept relatively general and cannot be used exactly as they are presented for everyone. Instead, they are intended to be guides as to which and how much training should be done. One person may have more time and enthusiasm than another, one person may need to train harder than another, and people's goals may be very different. There are many factors that may influence the training plan, which shows how hard or even impossible it is to draw up a one-size-fits-all training plan even for a single category. Individuality is essential. This book would have to be 500 pages long and contain a bewildering number of plans to cover all circumstances. The book cannot present the training plan, it just aims to help you orient yourself and provide the knowledge to set up your own training plan. Yet again, the training principles you use to set up your own training plan are important.

Bicycle tour riders and recreational cyclists

The main priority of bike tour riders and recreational athletes is to have fun and keep fit, with competitive ambitions usually taking a back seat. Men and women, children and adolescents all participate in bike tours, making them an ideal family sport.

Training is determined by the goals of the recreational cyclist, which can be divided into different groups: 1) occasional cyclist, 2) regular bike rider, and 3) bicycle tour riders who take their hobby very seriously and achieve peak performances in their sport. The bike tour rider, just like the racing cyclist, often rides in different tours every weekend during the season. Socializing with like-minded people and friends as well as the joy of movement are the priorities. Racing cyclists are often ignorant of the performances achieved by hobby cyclists.

The **occasional cyclist** doesn't need to abide by any strict plan; he just rides when he feels like it. However, he should not just rest during the winter but keep active by playing team games or running. In spring, he can start with short rides that gradually become longer as the season progresses. Should you want to go on a cycling holiday, you will definitely need to train more beforehand, otherwise a nice relaxing trip could turn into a painful ordeal. The occasional cyclist will cover almost 100% of his mileage in the BE 1 zone so as to be able to obtain maximum health benefits from his sport.

Bike tour rider

Km covered annually	5,000-10,000 km	10,000-15,000 km	15,000-20,000 km
Number of bike tours	10-20	20-30	30-50
Max. training distance	Up to 150 km	Up to 180 km	Up to 200 km
Training zones	BE 1, BE 2, RSE	BE 1, BE 2, RSE, (SE)	BE 1, BE 2, RSE, SE
Tips	• A lot of technique training	• Important: practice other sports	• Important: stretching exercises

Weekly cycles in PP and RP (10,000-15,000 km)

	PP	RP
Monday	Stretching, exercices, strengthing exercises	Swimming 500 m or as long as you want
Tuesday	30-50 km BE 1 or run (30-60 min)	40-60 km BE 1 2 km SE
Wednesday	Stretching, exercises strengthening exercises, other sports	30-50 km BE 1/2 Stretching, strengthening exercises
Thursday	Other sports or 30 km BE 1	50-80 km BE 1
Friday	Swimming 500-1.000 m	30 km CT/BE 1 or other sports
Saturday	30-60 km BE 1 or MTB	Bike tour 50-150 km
Sunday	Up to 80 km BE 1 or MTB	Bike tour 50-150 km

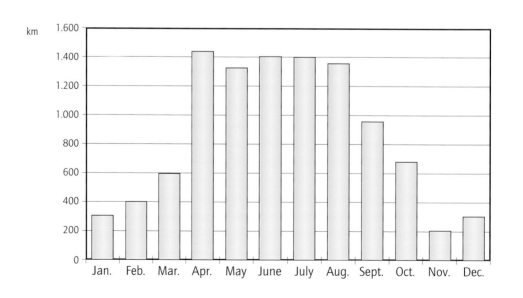

A **touring biker** spends considerably more time in the saddle of his two-wheeled friend (2,000-8,000 km) and occasionally takes part in a bike tour. Over the course of the year, training should, as mentioned, increase gradually, and in summer you can even occasionally ride at higher intensities.

The **bicycle touring cyclist** covers between 6,000 and 20,000 km every year and tries to get as fit as possible given the amount of training he does. The very conscientiously training and ambitious bike tour rider should base his training plan on that of junior cyclists, with a reduction in the speed and speed strength areas. Some bike tours resemble time trials or races. With low training intensities, performance levels can very often be significantly improved.

Balance is important

For all three groups, it is important to bear in mind that, particularly later in life, a one-sided cycling-only sporting activity may lead to problems with the musculoskeletal system (back). For this reason, along with cycling, another one or two different sports should be practiced in order to avoid any imbalances. As this usually affects more senior cyclists, a targeted muscle training for backs, arms, and abs as well as stretching exercises to improve flexibility are highly recommended (see chapter 3.9).

In this way, aches and pains in the musculoskeletal system can be prevented or at least alleviated. Regular medical checks with stress-ECG should be part of the routine of the health-conscious cyclist, as should a sports-appropriate diet.

Therapeutic cyclist

The therapeutic cyclist is not interested in competitive success; his primary goal is to do something for his health, be it preventive or rehabilitative. Exercise in the beautiful countryside and with friends adds to the recreational value of the sport. Cycling is actually preferable to running as a therapeutic sport, as it is low-impact and the exercise intensity is easier to control than in running. Higher speeds can be attained and longer rides can be full of variety. The relatively long distances covered enable riders to experience nature in all its glory along the way.

Cycling is ideal for those suffering from obesity or arthritis. Unfortunately, cycling is less popular as a therapeutic activity than group activities like team games or hiking, since cycling usually takes place in road traffic and the different performance levels within a group would mean that they would not be able to stick together. For therapeutic cyclists, the intensity must remain in the BE 1 and CT zones, because this category can often be a risk group that should not train too intensively. A rule of thumb assumes an exercise heart rate of 180 minus age, which usually comes out at around 130. High strength loads that involve blood pressure spikes (hills) must be avoided. Great importance should be attached to variety. Stretching exercises and other suitable sports like volleyball, Nordic walking, running, and swimming can be introduced into the exercise program. The therapeutic cyclist should undergo a medical check-up before taking up any sport.

Race Categories

The reader should read the plans for all categories as many basic issues and tips are scattered among the sections on each category and not repeated in every chapter. The women's racing categories are attached to the men's and features specific to women's training are noted.

U11 and U13

The youngest age groups are divided into two categories for both boys and girls: U11 and U13. It is quite possible for boys and girls to compete against each other in these categories. Often, girls are better than boys of the same age. The rights and wrongs of cycle racing for still such relatively young children, sometimes involving them sacrificing part of their childhood, are open to debate. Those concerned are often children whose parents push them into cycling and confuse their own ambitions with those of their children.

Young athletes should be treated very carefully, as errors committed when practicing sports and bad experiences can ruin children's enjoyment of sport and exercise for the rest of their lives. At club level, very sensitive and specially trained coaches and instructors are required. The danger of forcing precocious development in children is great. The drop-out problem is common in cyclists who took up the sport very early. This concerns athletes who no longer want to continue with the sport when they reach adulthood, thereby missing out on the most important phase of the sport from a competitive point of view. Parents should think very carefully and weigh whether they want to allow their children to compete in races at such a young age.

U 13

Age	11 (m)	12 (m)	11 (w)	12 (w)
Km covered annually	2,000-3,000 km	3,000-4,000 km	2,000-3,000 km	3,000-4,000 km
Number of races	5-10	Up to 15	5-10	Up to 15
Max. training distance	Up to 50 km	Up to 70 km	Up to 50 km	Up to 70 km
Training zones	BE 1, BE 2, (RSE), (ST)	BE 1, BE 2, (RSE), (ST)	BE 1, BE 2, (RSE), (ST)	BE 1, BE 2, (RSE), (ST)
Tips	• Make training varied	• Practice other sports	• As much technique training	• Only race infrequently

Weekly cycles in PP and RP (age 12)

	PP	RP
Monday	Other sports or rest	Other sports or rest
Tuesday	Indoor training 1 hr	30 km or ball game, technique training
Wednesday	Rest	Other sports
Thursday	Indoor training 1-2 hrs	30-50 km BE 1 with RSE sections for fun
Friday	Ball games 1 hr or rest	15 km CT / BE 1 + 2
Saturday	30 km BE 1 or MTB	30-50 km BE 1 + 2
Sunday	30-45 km BE 1 or MTB	Race or 30-60 km BE 1

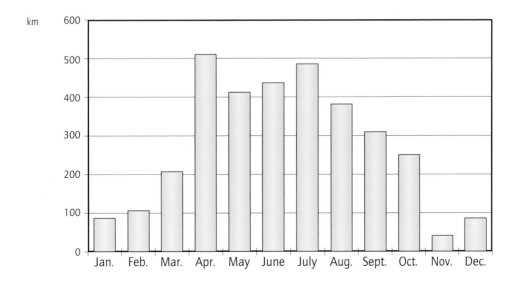

Cycling in moderation

However, the previous section was not meant to encourage a ban on all racing, as in moderation and with the right coaching, competition has a very positive effect on the young cyclist's mental and physical development. In the U13 age groups and other categories even up to junior level, there are considerable developmental differences between participants. Early, late, and normal developers from two cohorts have to compete against each other, with the result that the outcomes of races are often obvious in advance due to the huge differences in performance levels of the competitors. It is therefore necessary to distinguish between biological and calendar ages. There has been a definite tendency in recent decades for the biological age to run ahead of the calendar age (*accelerated development*).

In training for the under-13 category, the emphasis is on all-round sporting activity and must be structured in a child-friendly way, never according to adult training principles, which would make it too hard and monotonous.

More than in any other age group, cycling for kids should primarily be about having fun and enjoying the sport. Alongside bike training (approx. 50%), children should also acquire a general athletic foundation (running, swimming, games), for which team games and ball games are an excellent choice. Team games should take precedence as they promote social development and the acquisition of new movement experiences. On the bike, road safety and technique training must be given, and a helmet is compulsory for kids and all other age groups and with time will become second nature.

Sitting position

Growth spurts make it essential to regularly check and, if necessary, adjust children's sitting positions. In order to protect the growing body from excessive loads, gear ratios are limited in all age groups under the age of 19. For those in the U13 category, this is uniformly reduced to 5.66 m for every crank turn.

Training should lay the foundations for later high-performance cycling, and this is primarily achieved by basic endurance training. Faster sections and sprints are included for variety, but strength, speed, and interval training must be completely avoided. Rides should usually be about 30 km long on a course that is easy for children to cope with. A fixed, relatively traffic-free circuit should be used. Cyclists under 13 can do up to 70-km long low-intensity rides in the summer. Training is almost all carried out with the small wheel. Younger cyclists should not start regular road training until March. Before this, they should only train on the racing bike in nice, mild weather and focus on other sports. Young cyclists can compete in up to 15 races. Training for boys and girls is roughly the same at this age.

U15

In this age group, boys' and girls' training is generally the same, although the girls' volume may be slightly reduced. Race distances are usually around 20 km, with road races sometimes being up to 40 km. The basic comments about high-performance sport for children from the previous section are also valid for older children in this and the next age group. The under-15 age group is best time to take up cycling and try out a few races.

Keeping the number of races to a moderate level at a young age preserves motivation for high-performance training later on. This is why not more than 10-20 races per season should be entered. Unfortunately, it is not uncommon to see kids racing 35-40 times per season so that they spend the majority of their weekends in the car traveling to races. The enthusiasm of these children's ambitious parents must be restrained. Children's personality development must always take precedence over performance development and parents' desire for success.

More cycling training

A higher percentage (60-70%) of overall training is also done on the bike. As well as non-specific general indoor training in winter and in summer, one to two different sports are also practiced. It would be great if during the season, cycling clubs would offer a weekly general athletic training session combined with team games. Particular importance must be given to working on those parts of the body (arms, upper body) that are not used much in cycling. Mondays or Wednesdays are good days for this in the under-15 age group.

The transition phase with reduced cycling and general training can be prolonged to the end of November in this age group. In the preparation phase, do a lot of running and swimming. In no age group is it acceptable to think that little bike training equates to little or no training at all. Low-volume and low intensity bike training only resumes in February.

It is not necessary for those in the U15 category to start their season before the middle of April, and the end of the season can also be brought forward (to the middle of September), thus reducing the pressure on the young cyclists. This also means that any bad weather in March, April, and also in the fall can be avoided. During the racing season, most training is in the BE 1 and BE 2 zones. For under-15s and those new to cycling, more time is spent on BE 2 zone training than in the older age groups. Strength training is still prohibited, sprints (e.g., 6 point-to-point sprints) and RSE training (e.g., 3 x 1 km tempo) do belong in the training plan and should be performed in the middle of the week.

U15

Age	13 (m)	14 (m)	13 (w)	14 (w)
Km covered annually	4,000-6,000 km	5,000-7,000 km	3,000-5,000 km	4,000-6,000 km
Number of races	10-15	Up to 20	10-15	10-15
Max. training distance	Up to 100 km	Up to 120 km	Up to 80 km	Up to 100 km
Training zones	BE 1, BE 2, RSE, ST	BE 1, BE 2, RSE, ST	BE 1, BE 2, RSE, ST	BE 1, BE 2, RSE, ST
Tips	• Make training varied	• Practice other sports	• As much technique training as possible	

Weekly cycles in PP and RP (ages 13-14)

	PP	RP
Monday	Other sports or rest	Other sports or rest
Tuesday	20 km BE 1 or indoor training 1 hr	30-40 km with 3-5 sprints, technique training
Wednesday	Other sports or rest	30 km BE 1 or other sports
Thursday	Indoor training 1-2 hrs	40-60 km Be 1 with tempo intervals (BE 2, RSE)
Friday	Other sports 1 h or rest	15 km CT/BE 1 or rest
Saturday	30-50 km BE 1 or MTB	Race or 30-60 km BE 1 + 2
Sunday	30-60 km BE 1 or MTB	Race or 30-90 km BE 1

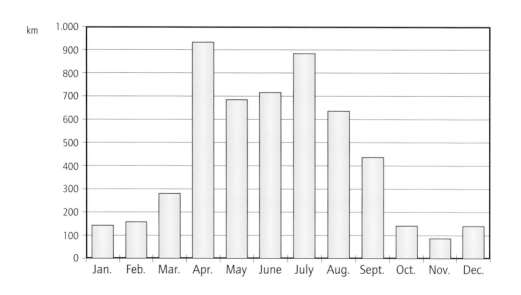

A lot of cycling technique

Cycling technique should not be neglected, particularly by newcomers to cycling. Technique training should be made fun. Ideal training distances are from 30-50 km on quiet, undulating courses. In the preparation phase, training distances may extend to 20-40 km, and cyclists in good physical shape can also do bike tours up to 80 km or even 120 km with longer rest breaks. In these cases, it is crucial that they do not try to keep up with adults but compete at an appropriate speed for their age (not alone on long rides). This, incidentally, is a very big problem, as under-15s commonly train with older cyclists (e.g., juniors or even amateurs), which not infrequently represents a total physical overload and often leads to frustration and lack of motivation. The times when it was thought that this aided the development of young cyclists are long gone. Not everything that is hard also makes you stronger. That is true in the most general sense for any weaker cyclists who train with significantly stronger ones as they tend to overextend themselves in training.

Precisely planned technique training is not strictly essential for under-14s; instead cyclists should train within set limits (volume) according to how they feel, while bearing in mind the points mentioned.

U17

In the U17 age group, boys compete in races up to 80 km and girls up to 60 km. Circuit races are usually 40 km for boys and are often held as criteriums.

There is a big jump from the U15 age group (where the cycling speed is usually still really slow) to the U17 age group. This is particularly true for the still small and slight late developers who must now compete against 16-year-olds who may be up to four biological years older than them. This situation often leads to problems of motivation for newcomers to the U17 age group. A maximum gear ratio roll-out of 6.99 m allows for high speeds to be reached so that strength acquires more importance in the development of power.

U17

Age	15 (m)	16 (m)	15 (w)	16 (w)
Km covered annually	7,000-9,000 km	8,000-10,000 km	6,000-8,000 km	7,000-9,000 km
Number of race	20-30	Up to 35	15-20	Up to 25
Max. training distance	Up to 130 km	Up to 140 km	Up to 110 km	Up to 120 km
Training zones	BE 1, BE 2, RSE, ST	BE 1, BE 2, RSE, ST, SS, (SE)	BE 1, BE 2, RSE, ST	BE 1, BE 2, RSE, ST, SS, (SE)
Tips	• A lot technique training	• Careful SE and ST from age 16 and up	• Get used to greater volumes	• Important: practice sports other than cycling

Weekly cycles in PP and RP (ages 15-16)

	PP	RP
Monday	Other sports or rest	Other sports or rest or 20 km CT
Tuesday	30 km BE 1 or indoor training 1 hr	30-40 km with 3-7 sprints or 2 km SE (52 x 17), technique training
Wednesday	Other sports or 30 km BE 1	40-50 km BE 1 and other sport
Thursday	Indoor training 1-2 hrs	50-60 km BE 1 with tempo intervals (BE 2, RSE)
Friday	Other sports 1 hr or rest	20 km CT/BE 1 or rest
Saturday	30-60 km BE 1 or MTB	Race or 40-90 km BE 1 + 2
Sunday	30-90 km BE 1 or MTB	Race or 40-120 km BE 1

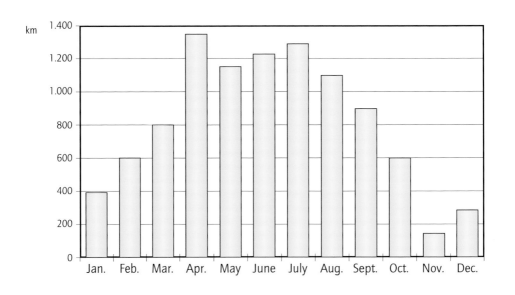

Starting strength training

The U17 age group is the time to start regular, structured strength training both on the bike and in the gym (with own bodyweight). The initial aim is not to increase maximal strength but to work with low weights and high repetitions. Correct movement execution and technique must be emphasized right from the start.

Great importance is attached to speed development in this age. Speed training should therefore be carried about once or twice a week, especially during the season. Speed and a smooth, efficient pedaling action are improved by using a high cadence in foundation training (around 90 rpm and above).

The training distance rises from 4,000-7,000 km in the previous age group to about 7,000-9,000 km in the first year and 8,000-10,000 km in the second year. Girls in this age group ride between 6,000-9,000 km per year.

Individual yearly training mileage

The training mileages recommended here for the year, month, or individual training rides are heavily dependent on the rider's objectives and time available for training, which should provide guidance as to training volume and content. However, the very top cyclists in most categories train more and sometimes even significantly more than this. But their training plans cannot be adopted by the average cyclist and more can often be achieved with less. Less ambitious cyclists naturally do less riding in training.

The aim of training in the U17 age group is to build a cycling-specific performance foundation that goes hand in hand with a significant increase in aerobic capacity. Furthermore, training should also include participation in a variety of other sports as well as cycling. It is still too soon to specialize in a single cycling discipline (e.g., cross-country or 500-m time trials on the track). For road-cycle racers in particular, track training comes as a welcome change that improves technique training. The same is true for mountain biking in the winter, which develops a feel for the bike. In technique training, more difficult techniques can now be introduced and advanced.

Juniors

Age	17 (m)	18 (m)	17 (w)	18 (w)
Km covered annually	10,000-13,000 km	12,000-16,000 km	8,000-10,000 km	10,000-13,000 km
Number of races	30-40	30-45	20-30	25-35
Max. training distance	Up to 160 km	Up to 180 km	Up to 130 km	Up to 150 km
Training zones	BE 1, BE 2, RSE, ST, SS, SE	BE 1, BE 2, RSE, ST, SS, SE	BE 1, BE 2, RSE, ST, SS, SE	BE 1, BE 2, RSE, ST, SS, SE
Tips	• SE and strength training become important	• Get used to high volumes	• Road races, a circuit	• Don't forget to practice other sports

Weekly cycles in PP and RP (ages 17-18)

	PP	RP
Monday	Other sports or rest	Other sports or rest or 30 km CT
Tuesday	30 km BE 1 Indoor training 1-2 hrs/strength training 1 hr	50-80 km with 5-8 sprints or 2-4 km SE (52 x 15), technique training
Wednesday	30-60 km BE 1 or run 1 hr	60-90 km BE 1 with 3 x 5 km RSE or training race
Thursday	Indoor training 1-2 hrs	80-130 km BE 1 with a few tempo intervals (BE 2, RSE)
Friday	Other sports 1-2 hrs or rest	30 km CT/BE 1 or rest
Saturday	40-70 km BE 1 or MTB Use weekend for 2-day block of BE training	Race or 60-150 km BE 1 + 2 If no race: BE-Block
Sunday	70-120 km BE 1 or MTB Use weekend for 2-day block of BE training	Race or 80-180 km BE 1 If no race: BE-Block

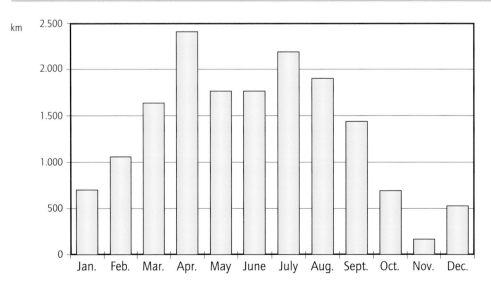

Heart rate training

Training should now be managed by using a heart rate monitor if this has not already started in the previous age group. The purpose of heart rate-oriented training should be explained to the cyclist and backed up by theory. Boys and girls in this age group train almost throughout the whole winter with the bike, and 80% of their training mileage is in the BE zones. Strength endurance training is started in April, while speed training is on the program from January onward. During the season, sprint training is done (e.g., 5-7 reps). The all-important general athletic training session with exercises and games is continued throughout the summer. During the in-season, between 20 and 30 or at most 35 races are contested.

Juniors

Cycling starts to get serious from the junior age group on. Young men and women 17 to 18 years old need to train hard just to be able to be competitive in races, let alone finish in the top three. Almost no other sport requires such high training volumes as cycling in all age groups, which is hard to understand and often frustrating for newcomers to the sport (i.e., those who have previously practiced ball games). Young athletes who take up cycle racing in the junior age group with no previous endurance sport experience, never mind at competitive level, find it extremely hard to cope with this. Often the first season comes and goes without them being able to compete in a single race. However, there are always very talented exceptions to this rule.

Unfortunately, familiarization races, which would gradually introduce cyclists to real races, are very rarely organized.

No performance categories

For organizational reasons, performance categories that would make the sport more accessible are also thin on the ground in the U19 age group.

Coaches and parents must be very understanding about this special situation that doesn't really arise in other sports to avoid demotivating the young cyclists. Instead, they should be encouraged to tackle the high training loads.

For those who have experience racing in previous age groups now begins the training phase in which the foundation is laid for a successful amateur career. For this reason, coach and cyclist should not lose sight of their long-term goals (for amateurs or women's categories). It is very tempting at this time to train so hard in order to achieve early successes that it is impossible to increase training in later years. The long-term build-up of the young cyclist must be respected.

Although yearly training volumes of 20,000 km for second-year juniors are sometimes recommended, for 95% of cyclists this is completely unrealistic. First they are still in school and do not have unlimited time available, and second, they still have other interests apart from cycling. It is quite possible to achieve top performances with yearly training volumes of 10,000-16,000 km for men and 8,000-13,000 km for women. With a well-constructed training plan, this can even be achieved with considerably less than 14,000 km per annum.

Fit in the winter

After a transition phase of six to eight weeks until the beginning to middle of November, systematic training starts for juniors in the gym, on the bike, and occasionally in the weight room. Regular running training until about the end of January should also enable training to be carried out on cold, damp days. Particularly before indoor training in the gym, which involves a lot of running and jumping still in the transition phase, cyclists must get used to the running action with a few runs in the forest (less than1 hr) in order to avoid injury problems and overloading symptoms especially in the lower limbs. Running on the roads should be avoided at all costs.

The emphasis of training in the preparation phase with its microcycles is on the continual improvement of aerobic capacity by means of basic endurance training. Coordination, strength, flexibility, and speed are improved by indoor training and practicing other sports. The very low training mileage in the months of December and January absolutely do not mean that the cyclist is not training; instead, he is improving his basic endurance with other endurance sports and in addition he still rides his bike.

Training camps for juniors

A training camp with very high training volumes in March or April (spring break) brings the preparation phase to a close. Depending on how much training has been done prior to the camp and what time of year it takes place, the training camp can also be used to build race-specific form. Generally for reasons of time, this is the only place where young cyclists can complete the very high training volumes that are essential for good form.

For very good juniors, training periodization leading to one important race (regional, national or even world championships) is recommended. Age 17 or 18 is a good time to specialize in one cycling discipline in which you are very successful or find most enjoyable. However, this specialization should not be taken to extremes, and other disciplines should also be contested.

Improve weaknesses

As well as the previously mentioned improvement of already very well-developed partial areas of the performance (sprint, climbing), individual weaknesses should also already be improved in juniors. A weak sprinter should carry out more sprint training, and a good sprinter who is poor at climbing should work on this aspect of his performance. From mid-February onward, sprint and strength endurance training should be introduced and each carried out once a week. Race-specific endurance is improved on Wednesdays or Saturdays with short intervals (3 x 3 km) with really easy gear ratios (52 x 17).

In the racing phase, May in particular is characterized by frequent racing; in this phase it is also important to do as many long road races as possible in order to build fitness. Also in the racing phase, about 70-80% of training kilometers are done in the basic endurance zones. Strength, sprint, speed, and also RSE training are included in the weekly training cycle. Cyclists should not forget to include a whole-body team game like soccer as well as stretching and strengthening exercises.

Strength training in the weight room is carried out once a week during the season. Roughly 30-45 races can be contested in the racing season. It is a good idea to enter training races during the week, particularly at the start of the racing phase. The summer holidays are a good time to do very long rides on a kind of home-based training camp.

High training volume

In the preparation phase, the longest basic endurance 1 rides in the men's category should not exceed approximately 120 km, and in the women's approximately 90 km. In the racing phase and at the end of the preparation phase (training camp), distances of up to 180 km in the case of young men, and young women should not exceed 150 km. In order to avoid overtraining, particularly on long rides, it is important to keep the intensity low (BE 1). In general, the basic rule is that the longer the training ride, the lower the intensity should be. Avoid very long rides of 150-180 km with average speeds of over 30 km/h as they do not lead to the desired training effect; a 25-28 km/h pace is quite sufficient. Young cyclists must be restrained in the mountains, otherwise their ambition can too easily lead to overloading.

Junior women ride proportionately less, and the training of first-year junior women should be based on that of first-year U17 boys.

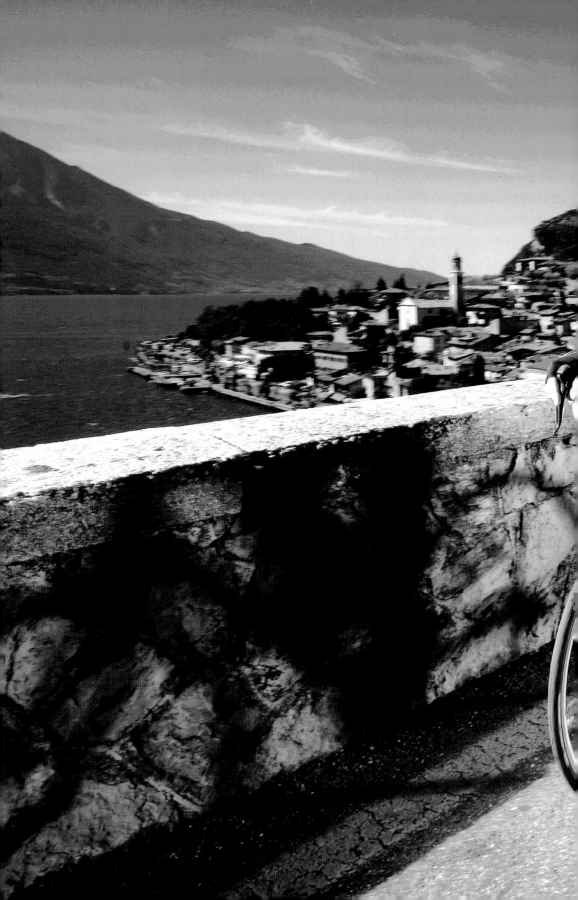

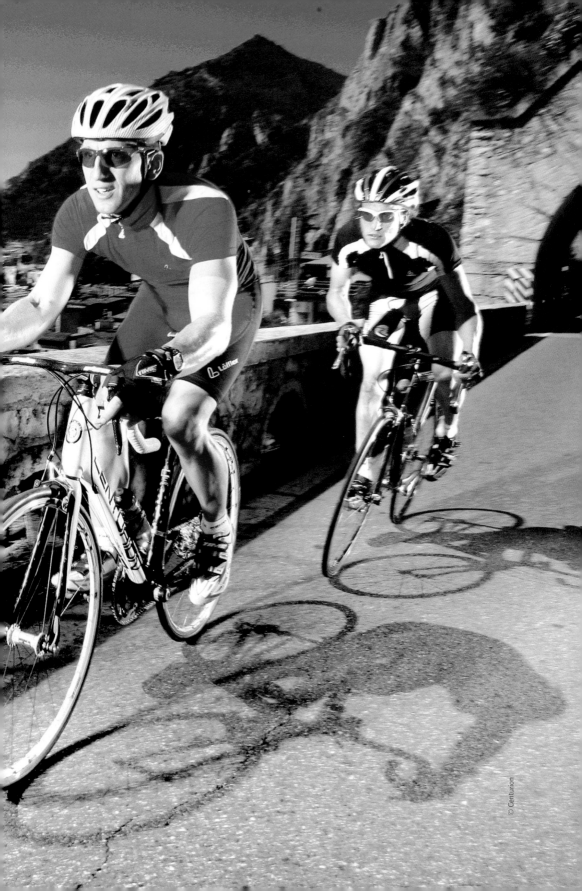

Lower amateur class and the first year

This category has the highest number of starters. To get up to higher categories, an exceptional performance is needed in terms of endurance, tactics and technique. This category comprises young amateurs who have advanced from the junior age group, cyclists who have been relegated from category 3, and amateurs who have been starting in category 5/4 for years. In addition, there are complete newcomers who understandably have a difficult time competing in this category, as well as masters who occasionally try to race with the amateurs again, sometimes with great success.

Different prerequisites

It would be impossible to provide training plans for such a disparate group. Cyclists' goals range from just enjoying the racing atmosphere to winning as many prizes as possible and not just rising through the categories but getting to category 1 as fast as possible. It is therefore important to set achievable goals and set your own training plan derived from the principles of the other racing categories. You must train according to certain principles and bear in mind the worst training errors and avoid committing them yourself.

Continuity

Former junior cyclists hoping to rise through the ranks from categories 5 (for men) and 4 (for women) must take a long-term view of their training and performance development. In their first amateur year, the yearly training distance increases to 14,000-16,000 km, which is achieved primarily through higher volumes in the preparation phase. In the racing phase, if possible, two to three smaller circuits (stage races) should be entered. Racing becomes a priority again. There is no question that even with lower training volumes it is possible to move up to the next category and that a few cyclists must train more than this. This particularly applies to the absolute top cyclists, who in any case have different goals and also compete in long and tough races. High training volumes are for those attempting to reach category 1 where competition is much tougher than in the lower categories.

In theory, in the first four amateur years, the annual training distance should increase by 2,000-4,000 km each year. However, this is only possible for those whose main activity is training and who do not have to work. So the annual training distance for most higher-category cyclists is around 20,000 km. The other training areas also increase proportionately during this process.

More races

There should be a sharp increase in the number of races, meaning strength endurance training should decrease. The racing density increases in the lower amateur categories to 40-60 races per season. For more ambitious cyclists, the long road races are the most important, and circuit races or criteriums should only rarely be contested. Because most tough races are decided in the mountains, mountain-cycling performance is key for long road races and circuits. Young amateurs must bear this in mind and train specifically for it (strength endurance). Reducing body fat and weight improves cycling performance both in the mountains and also in general. Basic endurance rides can exceed 200 km.

Don't make training errors

In the lower categories, there are an amazing number of cyclists who complete over 20,000 km of training per year but who have no success at all to show for it. How is this possible? As already mentioned in the section on training errors, these cyclists have no idea, or a completely wrong idea, of how to periodize their training and often their training intensity is too high. One feature of these cyclists is that during the year their performances remain pretty constant; in other words, their form is almost as good in the winter as it is in the summer. The monotonous, over-intensive training makes performance improvement impossible. These cyclists must radically rethink their approach to training and change it. By keeping the same training volume but structuring it correctly, performance will improve dramatically. If the excessive training volume of 20,000 km is significantly reduced and training is correctly structured, these cyclists can achieve at least the same performance levels as before the training restructure.

Basic endurance is the foundation

In all categories and zones, there must always be a foundation of basic endurance that is as well-developed as possible upon which to construct specific conditioning abilities. If the basic endurance level is inadequate, race-specific training usually leads to a drop in performance. With the right training, the late physical developer can catch up and often even overtake the early developer in the amateur category.

The typical lower-category amateur cyclist who would like to finish on the podium should be in a position to do so with an annual training volume of 12,000-14,000 km. The suggested training plan for the junior category will, in most cases, be quite adequate and lead to good performances.

In the case of a longstanding lack of success, very often the intensity must be reduced and periodization introduced. Increased importance should also be given to strength and speed training. Tactics must typically be reviewed or changed. Mental blocks are covered in detail in chapter 7. However, the large number of different cycling goals makes it impossible to create one standard training plan.

Top amateurs and U23

Races for these categories vary between 70-200 km. Most circuit races tend to be between 80-110 km, and road races range from 120-180 km. The longer racing distance, especially that of road races, necessitates harder training than in the lower amateur categories.

Yearly volumes of 15,000 km for category 2 and 3 amateurs and up to 40,000 km for the very top amateurs are required. An average top amateur should be able to cope with 20,000 km, although some cyclists need less but still compete successfully. The biggest problem in these categories is that here semi-professionals who can devote all their time to cycling and cyclists who are in employment or education compete against each other and are measured by the same standard. In addition, more and more races take place in which top amateurs must compete with all categories of professionals. In general, only continental European team professionals are admitted to top amateur races.

Even more racing miles

The proportion of racing kilometers increases significantly as races become longer and more frequent. Annually cyclists contest races that are between 40-100 km, some of which are circuit races. All training zones increase, and particular emphasis is placed on strength endurance, high race-specific endurance, and, as mentioned, on the greater number of races. Higher gear ratios and more mountain sections increase the importance of strength endurance. This is trained throughout the year until the transition phase—less at the start and end of the preparation phase and increased in the racing phase. Speed training is less important for road-racing cyclists. Basic rides should exceed 100 km and can even extend to 250 km. See the previous table for details of periodization. In the top amateur categories, training from the second preparation cycle on and during the season consists almost entirely of specific training on the bike; general athletic training is reduced to strength training (1-2 workouts per week) due to time constraints. However, an alternative sport should also be practiced during the season to provide a mental and physical break from cycling. Daily functional strengthening and stretching exercises attain an often-underestimated importance for high-performance cyclists.

Amateur U 23

	19 (m)	20 (m)	21 (m)	22 (m)
Age				
Km covered annually	16,000-20,000 km	20,000-24,000 km	22,000-26,000 km	24,000-28,000 km
Number of races	40-60	45-65	50-70	50-70
Max. training distance	Up to 200 km	Up to 250 km	Up to 250 km	Up to 250 km
Training zones	BE 1, BE 2, RSE, ST, SS, SE	BE 1, BE 2, RSE, ST, SS, SE	BE 1, BE 2, RSE, ST, SS, SE	BE 1, BE 2, RSE, ST, SS, SE
Tips	• SE and strength training very important	• Get used to high volumes	• Road race, circuits	• Don't forget to practice other sports

Weekly cycles in PP and RP (ages 19-22)

	PP	RP
Monday	Other sports or rest	Other sports, stretching, 30 km CT
Tuesday	60 km BE 1 Indoor training 1-2 hrs/strength training 1 hr	70-120 km with 7-12 sprints 4-15 km SE (53 x 14)
Wednesday	50-80 km BE 1 or run/ski 1-2 hrs	80-140 km BE 1 with 3 x 8 km RSE or training race
Thursday	Indoor training 2 hrs	120-200 km BE 1 with tempo intervals (BE 2, RSE)
Friday	Other sports 1-2 hrs or rest	30 km CT/BE 1 or rest
Saturday	70-130 km BE 1 or MTB Use weekend for 2-day block of BE training	Race or 90-180 km BE 1 + 2 If no race: BE-Block
Sunday	80-160 km BE 1 or MTB Use weekend for 2-day block of BE training	Race or 80-180 km BE 1 If noch race: BE-Block

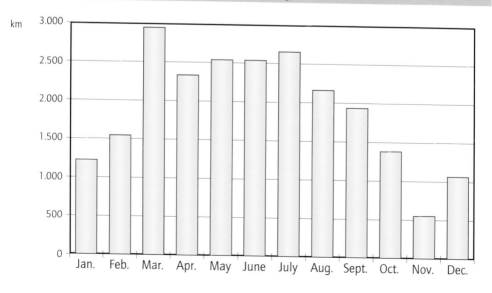

Strength training

Specific strength training using weights is organized according to the plan in chapter 3.8, Strength Training. A cyclist can only be as strong as his weakest link. For example, if the shoulder and arm muscles are very poorly trained, this prevents full performance development in climbing or sprints. If the abs and arm muscles are too weak, the body cannot develop the necessary tension for a vigorous acceleration or sprint and results remain average.

In addition, well-trained midsection muscles help protect the cyclists from overuse injuries. However, this doesn't mean that the cyclist should build up his muscles in the gym as they would just steal oxygen; instead you should improve the functionality of existing muscles.

Promotion

Young second-year amateurs should now focus on promotion through the categories. Those who have already achieved this should concentrate on big races. The requirement for increased cycling volumes of 10-20% per year is mainly met by longer races and circuits. It is a good idea to join a club that can enter teams in circuit races. The more performance levels improve, the more obvious it becomes that further performance improvement can only be achieved by increasing the racing mileage if the other training factors are correct—especially when the cyclist has no more time to spare for training.

A specific training method for amateurs is training behind a motorbike on quiet roads at very high speeds (racing speed or higher), taking advantage of riding in its slipstream. This type of training is a good race substitute and helps pace training, although it is not without its dangers.

Specialists

The top amateur categories are mainly populated by real circuit specialists and by road racers. While the former manage with low annual training volumes and only occasionally compete in road races in order to improve their basic endurance, the second group only occasionally compete in circuits and criteriums in order both to improve their speed and to attempt to win a share of the prize money. Road-racing cyclists should, if possible, contest very few circuit races and concentrate exclusively on long road races and circuits.

Women

The previous section is also largely true for amateur women. Races are roughly the same length as those in the junior men's category, and women may also enter junior races if no women's races are being held. As races are shorter, a lower annual training volume is also required, although in recent years this has risen sharply. For the first year in the amateur women's category, the cyclist should aim for a volume of 14,000 km. Top female cyclists complete an annual volume of 22,000-24,000 km.

Equality

As cycling is traditionally a man's sport, women have always had to fight for equality, which is still yet to be achieved in certain areas. After many years of discussion, people have finally realized that, particularly in endurance sports, women are capable of achieving almost the same performances as men. In cycling though, they are still relatively far from achieving this, which means that there is room for big performance improvement in the future. This would then mean that race distances would need to be longer, which has actually been happening gradually. However, men's races are still significantly longer.

Don't forget strength training

In the women's category, the emphasis is still on basic endurance training, which aids the development of high aerobic capacity. Historically, strength and strength endurance training have been, and still are, largely neglected by women, even though there is no doubt that they would significantly improve their performance. Strength endurance training is done with easier gear ratios and slightly reduced volumes compared to the amateurs. Female cyclists should pay particular attention to reducing their body fat proportion as much as possible. Those who naturally have little subcutaneous fatty tissue possess a clear advantage. They have a higher VO_2max, among other things.

Masters

Masters races are usually contested by former amateurs who still enjoy the excitement of cycle racing and want to continue to pursue the hobby they love with commitment. It is very rare to find newcomers to cycling in these age groups. These cyclists are usually very experienced and have excellent tactical ability.

Women

Age	19 (w)	20 (w)	21 (w)	22 (w)
Km covered annually	12,000-16,000 km	14,000-18,000 km	16,000-20,000 km	18,000-22,000 km
Numbers of races	25-40	30-45	35-50	35-50
Max. training distance	Up to 160 km	Up to 180 km	Up to 200 km	Up to 200 km
Training zones	BE 1, BE 2, RSE, ST, SS, SE	BE 1, BE 2, RSE, ST, SS, SE	BE 1, BE 2, RSE, ST, SS, SE	BE 1, BE 2, RSE, ST, SS, SE
Tips	• SE and strength training, very important	• Get used to highest volumes	• Road race, circuits	• Don't forget to practice other sports

Weekly cycles in PP and RP (ages 19-22)

	PP	RP
Monday	Other sports or rest	Other sports, exercices, 30 km CT
Tuesday	60 km BE 1 Indoor training 1-2 hrs/strength training 1 hr	60-100 km with 7-12 sprints 4-15 km SE (52 x 15)
Wednesday	40-70 km BE 1 or run/ski 1-2 hrs	60-120 km BE 1 with 3 x 8 km RSE or training race
Thursday	Indoor training 2 hrs	90-180 km BE 1 with tempo intervals (BE 2, RSE)
Friday	Other sports 1-2 hrs or rest	30 km CT/BE 1 or rest
Saturday	70-100 km BE 1 or MTB Use weekend for 2-day block of BE training	Race or 90-150 km BE 1 + 2 If no race: BE-Block
Sunday	80-130 km BE 1 or MTB Use weekend for 2-day block of BE training	Race or 90-180 km BE 1 If no race: BE-Block

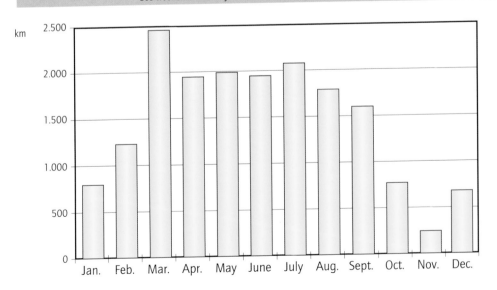

Short races

Overly short race distances that rarely exceed 50-60 km often meet with criticism. Large entries and short courses often lead to mass sprint finishes. However, longer races would be more suitable for more senior cyclists as longer races mean a lower intensity. During the course of their careers, most masters cyclists already have so many racing and training miles under their belts that they know exactly what is good for them and what is not. However, despite all traditional training wisdom, here, too, the emphasis should be on basic endurance training.

Balance is still important

It is very important to also practice a different sport (swimming, ball game) and to keep up the daily functional exercises that protect more senior competitive cyclists from overuse injuries and improper biomechanical stress. They also help maintain flexibility and coordination well into old age. The spine can be kept pain-free by means of specific spinal exercises. Widely differing goals and time availabilities make it impossible to provide meaningful sample training plans.

3.7   Training Camps

Why training camps?

Training camps in sunny climes, or even close to home, offer those cyclists who are usually busy working or studying the possibility of dedicating themselves completely to their sport for two or three weeks. The objective is a performance improvement that would be very hard to achieve by staying at home, otherwise it would be very difficult to cover such long distances in such a short period of time. A training camp in sunny climes is now firmly on the agenda of the preparation phase of most amateur cyclists. The different surroundings bring new motivation to the sometimes-monotonous preparation phase where training is always done in the same environment.

Training camp locations

Places with a daytime temperature of around 68-70°F or more are ideal for warm-weather training camps where training can be done in shorts. It is also possible to hold training camps closer to home in colder weather in order to toughen up for the spring classics and also to save money. Home-based training camps are also recommended for youth cyclists. However, the risk of catching a cold should be kept in mind and minimized by wearing the right clothing and eating a vitamin-rich diet. It is quite common to catch a cold in the initial weeks after returning home from warm-weather training camps.

When is the best time for a training camp?

As previously mentioned, training camps are usually held toward the end of the preparation phase. So for cycle racing, the most beneficial time is between the end of February and the end of March. For school children, the spring break is an ideal time, which is usually slightly later than this. Recreational cyclists can also go on warm-weather training camps in mid-March. It is even possible to hold skiing training camps in the winter. Elite cyclists also go on training camps during the season before important peak races. Altitude training camps are frequently used to give a vital boost.

Training camp duration

Two weeks seems to be the optimal length for most adults, while one week is sufficient for youth. However, elite cyclists' camps can last up to four weeks.

What kind of training is done in training camps?

That depends mainly on what kind of training has been done at home during the preparation phase. In a training camp at the end of February, the majority of training would definitely be basic endurance training, while in a training camp in April or during the season, the emphasis would be more on specific conditioning qualities involving fine-tuning fitness with specific, more intensive methods. It would make no sense to carry out intensive training in February when cyclists may not even have 2,000 km of training under their belts. In general, the training camp should be used for long training rides for which there is only rarely sufficient time at home. If a lot of training has been done already, intensive training phases (SE, RSE, ST) can be added. If cyclists are fit enough, they may also enter local races.

Three or four increasingly high-mileage days are followed by a CT day with a relaxed, two-hour ride. Then the next three- or four-day training cycle begins, this time with an even higher mileage than the previous one. More details can be found in the training plan for a two-week training camp. Strength endurance training should be included in every training plan in any case, and the higher the fitness level, the more strength training can be done (see table 3.2).

Table 3.2: Training camp for amateurs

	1st Week		2nd Week
1.	Arrive, 30-60 km warm-up	8.	180 km BE 1
2.	110 km BE 1	9.	2nd rest day, 50 km CT
3.	140 km BE 1 4 km SE	10.	140 km BE 1 15 km SE (z. B. 3 x 5 km)
4.	160 km BE 1	11.	160 km BE 1+2 some BE 2 sections
5.	1st rest day, 50 km CT	12.	180 km BE 1
6.	130 km BE 1+2 10 km SE	13.	220 km BE 1
7.	150 km BE 1	14.	Fly home poss. 30-50 km CT

Alternatives to cycling

Stretching and functional exercises should not be neglected. Early morning exercise is a challenge for many athletes. It is up to you to decide whether or not you need to do it. Ball games (e.g., table tennis, tennis, volleyball), when not played too intensively, add variety, and a balanced leisure program keeps boredom at bay. Take care with swimming though, as it is very easy for cyclists susceptible to colds to catch a chill and miss several days of training as a result. If you absolutely want to swim, reserve this for the final days of the camp. However, there is nothing to stop you enjoying hot relaxing baths or visits to the Jacuzzi or sauna.

Diet is important

During the training camp and also at home, great attention should be paid to the diet. Pigging out at the hotel buffet does not help you lose body fat, and many cyclists put on weight instead of losing it. However, do make sure you have an adequate, high-quality carbohydrate intake. Sufficient sleep is a prerequisite for successful training, as the high training volumes make long recovery times necessary. The two training plans below are suggestions for amateurs or juniors at two-week warm-weather training camps and for youngsters at home-based training camps. Both are mainly based on basic endurance training.

The suggested distances assume that a lot of training has already been done in the weeks prior to the training camp. During the two weeks, depending on fitness, category, and weather, cyclists should cover between 1,600 and 2,100 km. In the long daily rides, it is imperative to stick to the BE 1 zone, even though many mountains and a final sprint provide tempting opportunities to ride fast. Intensive training over such long distances would be excessive.

Table 3.3: Training camp for young cyclists

Day	Content
1.	Travel, 70 km BE 1, technique training
2.	80 km BE 1
3.	100 km BE 1
4.	50-70 km BE 1+2, technique + tactic training
5.	100 km BE 1+2
6.	110 km BE 1
7.	30-50 km, individual time trail (5 km), travel home

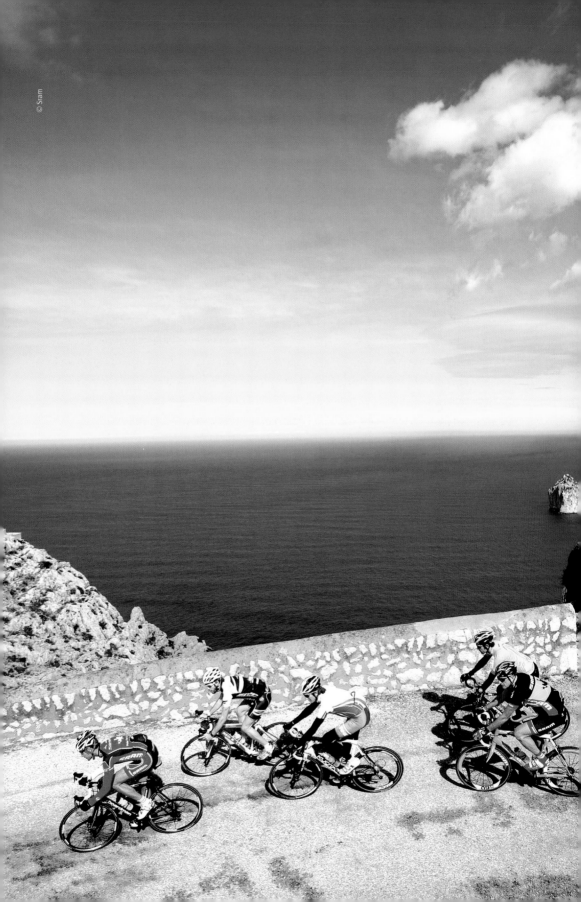

With the exception of the first cycle, strength endurance training takes place after each rest day with still relatively low volumes. For other categories, volumes must be reduced following the same principles. For logistical reasons, the daily volume can be done in two rides, although the long workout that completes the block should be done as a single workout.

3.8   Strength Training

In endurance sport in general and in cycling in particular, it took a long time for the importance of strength training to be recognized, and few elite athletes followed a planned strength training program, which even then was limited to the winter months. This situation reflected the belief that in endurance sports, strength levels had only a minimal effect on performance. However, it is now thought that strength plays an important role in developing endurance levels, and in cycling it enables cyclists to cope with high gear ratios.

This is one important reason why it should not be neglected, for if the strength to pedal at a particular gear ratio is lacking, even very good endurance levels are of little use. In ergometer tests, cyclists with good strength levels can maintain the required power for significantly longer than weaker cyclists. However, training science still lacks a consensus on how training should be done, although really good results can be obtained with the popular, more traditional methods.

A question of definitions

Uncertainty still reigns particularly when it comes to the definition of the different types of strength and their training methods, and the literature often contains contradictory advice. However, the methods and exercises presented here correspond predominantly to the current doctrine. According to more recent studies, maximal strength is much more important for the level of other types of strength (e.g., speed strength, strength endurance, explosive strength) and also for specific cycling performance than had previously been assumed.

Year-round training

Year-round strength training should be encouraged not only at elite level but for all cyclists, although with different goals. While at elite and competitive levels the aim is cycling-specific performance improvement; strength training for recreational cyclists is done for the purposes of injury prevention in order to provide protection from overuse injuries and improper biomechanical stress. This aspect should definitely not be neglected by elite cyclists, as specific training for the postural and supporting muscles (trunk, shoulders, arms) effectively prevents musculoskeletal injuries.

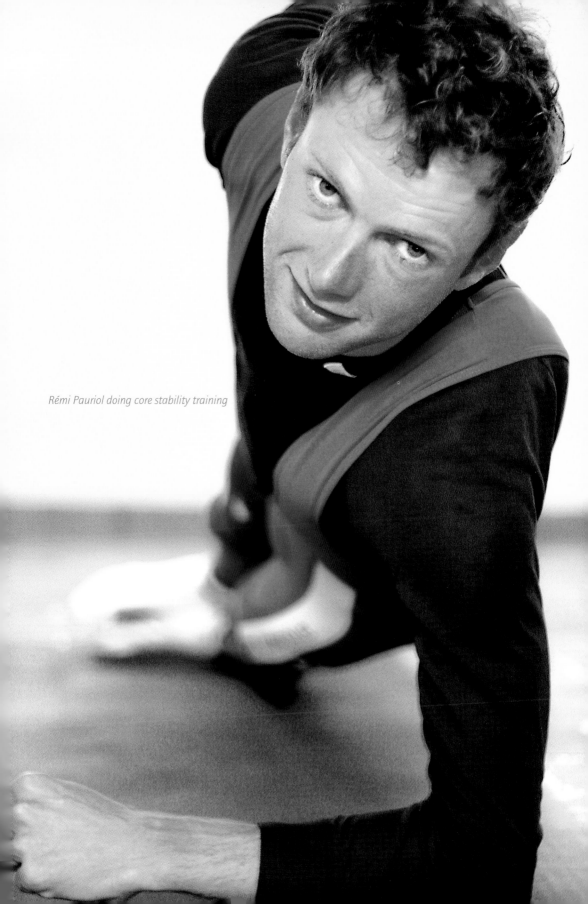

Rémi Pauriol doing core stability training

Improving muscle function

Strength training for cyclists definitely does not mean increasing muscle mass, but rather means improving the fitness levels of existing muscles, which only occasionally involves lifting weights. This functional improvement goes hand in hand with an increase in maximal strength and is done by improving the inter- and intra-muscular coordination of the muscles involved in a movement. Significant muscle cross-section enlargement (muscle growth) can only be achieved after long-term training with heavy weights, which in cycling should be avoided in most cases by specific training.

When to train?

Very often, strength potential that has been painstakingly developed in the preparation phase soon reverts to the starting level if it is not kept up during the season. Even regular strength training carried out once per week could maintain strength levels, thereby improving cycling-specific performance. Everything therefore points to riding a few miles less per week in order to use that time for strength training. For example, one hour every Wednesday before a gentle ride out on the roads is quite enough, and strength training can also be slotted in on bad weather days. The strength foundation is always laid in the weight room or in indoor training during the preparation phase.

As strength training is usually quite exhausting, and injuries can be caused by incorrect execution of the exercises, a few training rules and correct movement execution must be observed. In strength training for cycling, we differentiate between strength training in the gym or in the weight room (with machines or bodyweight) from strength training with the bike, which has already been comprehensively covered in chapter 3.3.

Strength training rules

- An intensive warm-up program must precede strength training, whatever form it takes. The higher the load, the longer the warm-up program should be.
- Just as in endurance training, strength training should follow the principle of gradual loading increase; only once a basic strength foundation has been laid can specific strength training begin.
- Strength training must be performed regularly (1-3 times per week).
- As in endurance training, the load must be varied and cyclized, as constantly training with the same load fails to trigger an adaptation process or associated training effect.
- Strength training must be adapted to performance level and age; before the age of 15, strength training should be limited to bodyweight exercises; overloading must be avoided.

- Correct and clean movement execution is essential (concentrate on the exercise).
- Breathe gently during the exercises, no forced exhalation.
- Remember the importance of recovery. Don't train when the body is exhausted after a race or hard workout; allow two to four minutes of rest between sets.

No specific numbers of reps and sets are given for the strength training exercises suggested next, as every athlete is different. It is better to choose the most suitable figures for you from the listed zones based on your training experience.

1   In the Weight Room

The weight training program given here covers the entire training year.

Determine maximum strength

The loading intensity is given as a percentage of maximum strength, which—after a thorough warm-up—must be tested on each machine or for each exercise separately in order to be able to calculate the percentages for the respective loads.

In a maximal strength test, take three or four attempts at your maximum weight. Make a note of the figures and use them to calculate your training program, and put it down in writing. A maximal test should be repeated roughly every month in order to adapt training loads to your improving strength levels.

The following muscle groups should be trained:

- **Thigh muscles** (hamstrings: different leg presses, squats with long bar, not too deep. quadriceps: different pulley machines, leg extension machine)
- **Lower leg muscles** (calf raise machine, toe raise with long bar)
- **Hip flexors**
- **Gluteal muscles** (see thigh)
- **Arm, shoulder**, and **chest muscles** (biceps curls, bench press, triceps curls, bench pull, lat pull-down, push-ups)
- **Back muscles** (back machine without weights, see chapter 3.8 on stretching, push-ups)
- **Abdominal muscles** (crunches, abs machine, abdominal exercises in chapter 3.9, push-ups)

You should have an experienced weight training instructor explain the provided exercises to you in a gym or weight room and combine them with exercises from the sections, Indoor training (page 117) and Stretching (chapter 3.9). A strength training session is composed of a warm-up section, a main section (always stretch between the exercises), and a cool-down. In the main section you should concentrate on training one or two muscle groups with several different exercises, alternating with back and abdominal exercises which should also be performed daily in your exercise routine.

Preparation periodization I (familiarization phase)
In November, strength training starts with low loads (45-55%) and high reps (15-20) in 2-4 sets in order to prepare the body for the more intensive training to come. This type of training should be done two to three times weekly in the weight room. It will be necessary to perform another maximal strength test after this phase.

Preparation periodization II (growth phase)
In December and in January, training weight increases to 60-70%, with 3-4 sets of 8-12 reps. As only two of these sessions are done weekly, there is no danger of developing excessively large muscles.

Preparation periodization III (maximal strength phase)
February and March are used for improving maximal strength (i.e., training weight is now very heavy (80-100%) with only 4-6 sets of 1-5 reps, leading to an increase in maximal and speed strength. Strength training should be done two or three times a week. Maximal strength should be checked several times during this period and training loads adjusted accordingly.

Racing periodization (strength maintenance phase)
In the racing phase from April onward, as mentioned previously the aim is to maintain strength levels by training one to two times weekly at 60-70% with 3 sets of roughly 8 reps. During the long racing phase, strength training loading must be varied just as the endurance loading is by occasionally adding a maximal strength workout, reducing training after tough races, and also varying the weight training exercises performed.

Table 3.4: Annual strength training program for cyclists

	Intensity	Reps	Sets	Session/Week
1. PP	45-55%	15-20	2-4	2-3
2. PP	60-70%	8-12	3-4	2-3
3. PP	80-100%	1-5	4-6	2-3
4. RP	60-70%	8	3	1-2

These 30- to 45-minute strength training sessions will allow you to maintain your strength during the season, enabling you to cycle more effectively (sprints, climbs, time trials) and maintain a smooth pedaling action with the high gear ratios that are essential to achieve good performances. In recreational and therapeutic cycling, strength training is limited to low weights and high reps (phase 1, possibly 2).

2   In the Gym or at Home

Effective strength training can also be done in the gym or at home, mainly with bodyweight exercises. When done correctly and in combination with strength training on the bike, it can re-place strength training in the weight room. Better still is a combination of strength training on machines and with free weights. There are two different main strength training methods that can be used in the gym or at home: dynamic and static training. It is important to not just do leg strengthening exercises, but also to include exercises for the arms, abs, back, and shoulders in your program (at elite level: whole-body training with the emphasis on the leg muscles; at grass-roots level: emphasis on the core muscles of the mid-section). A selection of strength training exercises for the gym are listed next, grouped according to part of the body.

What should be kept in mind?
The numbers of reps and sets should be adapted according to age, fitness, and goals so that a recreational cyclist would use the numbers of reps and sets at the lower end of the given range, while the trained elite cyclist would use the higher figures. If you train so hard that each time you suffer from severe muscle soreness, the weights are definitely too heavy; avoid muscle soreness or extreme exhaustion.

Legs

Calf muscles

Face the wall and stand on one ball of the foot, extend your ankle and then flex it again. Hold the other foot up or rest it against the heel of the active leg. It is important to straighten the knee of the active leg so that only the calf muscles perform the raising and lowering movement of the body. This exercise can be done even better on a step or a box. Do 2-4 sets of 15-50 reps.

Shin muscles

Sit on the floor with your legs stretched and flex your ankles by pointing your toes while keeping your heels on the floor. A partner exerts pressure on your toes. Do 2-4 sets of 10-20 reps.

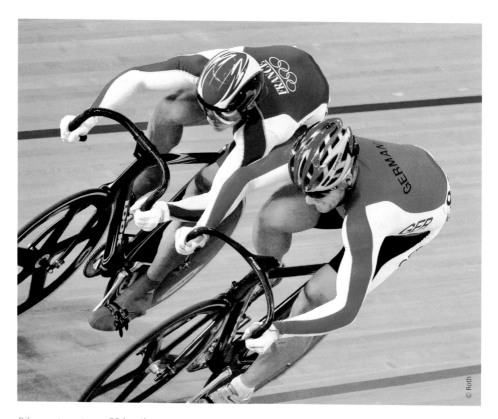

Bike mastery at over 60 km/h

Hamstrings, calves, and glutes

There is a whole series of strengthening exercises for the hamstrings:

1. Sit as if sitting on a chair and hold this position for 15-60 seconds. Keep your back straight and pressed against the wall and your arms down by your sides.

2. Depending on your fitness level, perform 10-30 two-legged crouch jumps over a bench (back and forth) for 2-4 sets.

3. Standing jump: Jump with both feet, keeping your back straight. After landing on flat feet, or better still on the balls of your feet, bend your knees no lower than an 80-degree angle and then take off again as quickly as possible. Complete 3-5 sets of 8-20 reps. This exercise is particularly good for improving climbing and sprinting performance. At elite level, this exercise can be made harder by jumping down from and up onto small boxes.

4. Almost all jumping exercises are suitable for strengthening the leg muscles, but one-legged jumps (hops) should only be performed if strength levels are high.

Jumping exercises, particularly exercises 2 and 3, improve speed strength. Jumping rope combines strength and endurance training and is therefore an excellent way of improving strength endurance. A program for the legs should always include a combination of several exercises.

Back, abs, arms, and shoulders

Exercises for these parts of the body can be found at the end of chapter 3.9, Stretching. Medicine ball training is a good option for the arm and shoulder muscles. In two sets, two cyclists throw a medicine ball back and forth to each other using different throwing and pushing techniques. A short strengthening program for the core and arm muscles should ideally be carried out daily in order to avoid overuse injuries.

On the bike

Strength training on the bike has already been covered in detail in chapter 3.8. A training form to improve the different types of strength and the anaerobic metabolism is repeated here: After a thorough warm-up (minimum 30 min), using sprint gear ratios perform 6 to 10 accelerations from an almost standing start as fast as possible for 30 seconds. Rest for 3-5 minutes by pedaling gently between each acceleration. For young cyclists, the duration should be reduced from 30 to 20 seconds with no more than 6 reps.

3.9 Stretching

What is stretching?

Stretching is a type of exercise that primarily impacts flexibility. Every athlete should carry out a daily stretching program, ideally combined with a few strengthening exercises as part of his training program. However, avoid stretching or only stretch after consulting a doctor in the case of injuries or after operations to the musculoskeletal system. Particularly for cyclists, stretching is an essential way of maintaining flexibility, as only the legs are moved in the cycling action and the rest of the body is neglected. The muscles shorten over time, which reduces flexibility and also the quality of the movement execution.

What does stretching achieve?

Stretching boosts the blood circulation and therefore the metabolism in the muscles, first preparing the muscles and tendons for the workout to come and then accelerating the post-exercise (training or racing) recovery. Stretching during warm-up reduces the risk of injury and makes for better muscle coordination and more efficient muscle function. A regular stretching program will reduce adhesions in muscle, tendon, and connective tissues, thus increasing muscle functionality. Muscle elasticity and the range of motion of the joints are significantly improved. A specific stretching program can even relieve troublesome muscle tension (e.g., in the back). Last but not least is another very important point: Stretching improves your physical awareness and perception; you get to know your body better and feel the slightest changes more quickly. It also just feels good, relaxes you, and is even fun. This long list of convincing arguments should definitely encourage you to start stretching.

How do you stretch?

There are a few points to bear in mind to ensure that you stretch correctly. The most important principle when stretching is that you concentrate on the stretched part of the body during the exercise in order to be aware of the sensations of tension and relaxation. During the 10- to 30-second stretching process (per exercise), you should feel a pleasant tension in the muscles that subsides slightly near the end of the exercise, at which point the tension can then be increased further. To start with you can even count out loud to measure the duration of the stretch, but as your sense of timing improves this will no longer be necessary.

You should not experience pain and grit your teeth when stretching. If the tension in the muscles is too great, reduce it slightly by changing the joint angles. Bouncing and jerking activate what is known as the **stretch reflex** and cause further cramping in the muscles. If a muscle is suddenly strongly stretched by bouncing or jerking, the muscle spindles are activated, leading to a sudden contraction of the muscle via the spinal cord. The stretch reflex protects a muscle from overstretching or tearing by intervening and contracting the muscle if it is overstretched.

Before the stretching program, you should warm up a little by continuous running in place, hopping, or riding on the roller (5 min). Breathing while stretching should be slow, regular, and controlled. Do not hold your breath as this could lead to forced breathing on exertion. Wear comfortable clothing (jogging suit) and if possible sit on a comfortable surface in a warmish room. Stretching on the bike should only be done on quiet roads or on a cycle path when you are in full control of the bike as you will need to perform a few contortions.

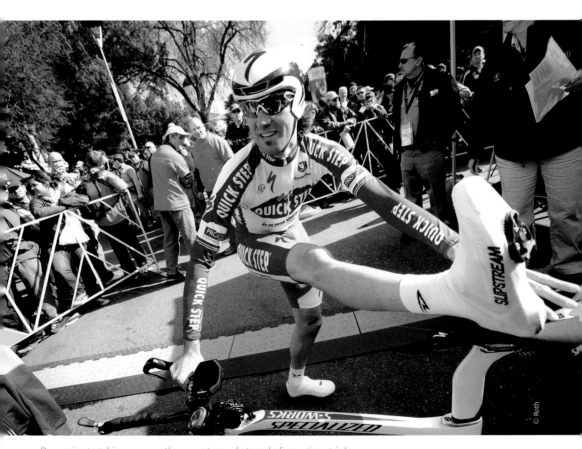

© Roth

Dynamic stretching ensures the correct muscle tone before a time trial.

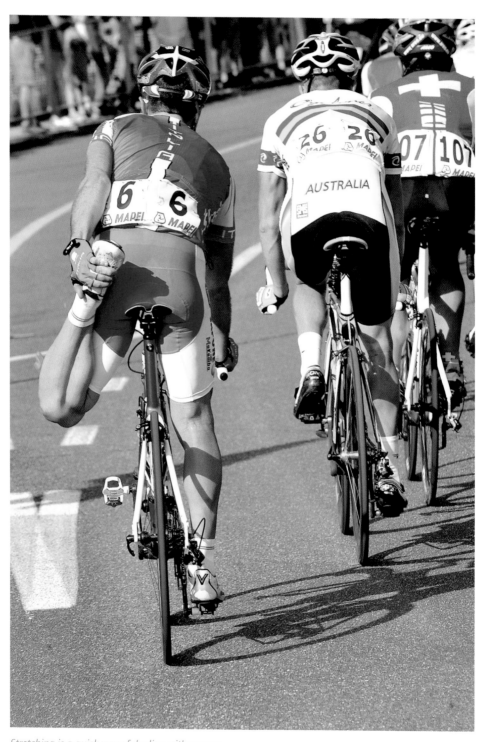

Stretching is a quick way of dealing with cramps.

Exercises on the bike

1. Neck

Hyperextending the neck when cycling often causes very painful muscle cramps.

Bend your head to the left and right for 5 seconds in each direction, or increase the stretch by pulling with one arm. Alternatively, round your back and place your chin on your chest, supporting the stretch a little with one arm by applying only very light pressure (be careful!). See illustration for exercise 1.

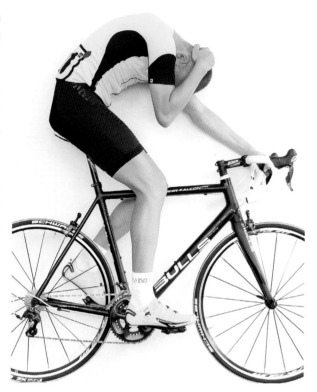

2. Spine/core

Ride with no hands, stretch out, and stretch your arms up to make yourself as tall as possible.

3. Shoulder girdle

With a narrow handlebar grip, straighten your arms, raise both shoulders to your ears (5 seconds) and then push them down. Next, take one hand off the handlebar, let your arm hang down loosely, and then move the whole arm in a circle a few times forward and backward.

4. Upper arm and shoulder

With the right hand on the handlebar, pass the left hand in front of the chin and place it on the right shoulder. Now move your hand around the shoulder toward the middle of the back as far as it will comfortably go. This stretches both the left triceps and shoulder.

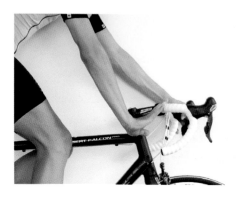

5. Hands and arms

With one hand on the handlebar, place the back of the other hand on your hip for 10 seconds until you can feel a stretch in the hand, forearm, and shoulder. This relaxes hands that are tired from gripping the handlebar. Wrist circling also increases the relaxation.

6. Back

Tense and aching backs require vigorous stretching.

    a. Holding the handlebar normally, first round then arch your back. Repeat both movements several times.

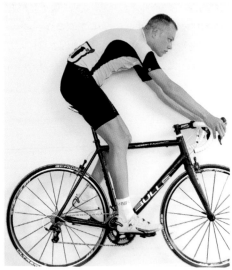

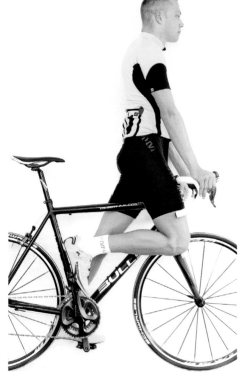

    b. While the left hand holds the handlebar, bring your right arm under your left arm so that the upper body twists as you stretch the core muscles (5-10 sec per side).

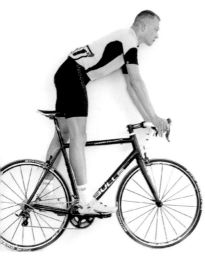

7. Hamstrings

The hamstrings can be stretched quite successfully on the bike. Lift yourself out of the saddle and bring the left pedal forward to the 9 o'clock position. Resting the balls of the feet on the pedals, lower your heels, straighten your legs, and bend your upper body forward (5-10 sec). Then repeat on the other leg.

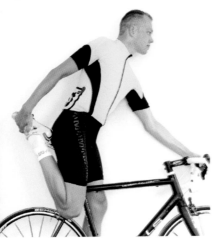

8. Quadriceps

The quads can also be stretched while cycling, although it does require a little riding expertise and good balance. Lift one foot off the pedal and grip the ankle with the same-side hand. Now pull the knee back slightly until you feel a stretch.

9. Calf and Achilles tendon

Raise yourself out of the saddle, and keeping the crank vertical, push the lower leg down. Push the heel of that leg down until you can feel a stretch. In order to transfer the stretch to the Achilles tendon, bend the knee of the straightened leg slightly.

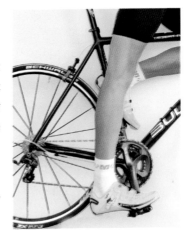

The last three exercises (7, 8, and 9) are suitable for eliminating troublesome cramps, particularly in the calves.

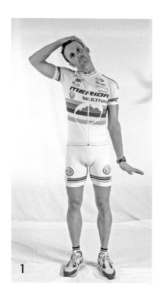
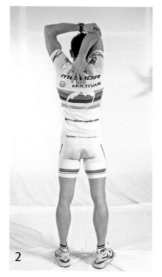
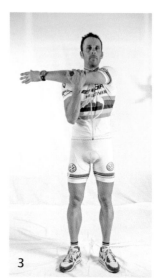

1   2   3

Pre-training, post–training, and racing exercises

1. Front and back neck muscles

Just as on the bike, the stretching program on terra firma starts with the head–neck area. Bend your head to the front, left, and right for 30 seconds each in order to stretch the neck muscles. The shoulders should remain horizontal throughout. Stretch the head as far as possible to the left and hold the position, then repeat to the right.

2. Shoulder

Circle the arms or shoulders to relax them. Stretch the shoulder girdle by bringing the elbows above the head and placing the palm of the hand between the shoulder blades. Hold this position for about 10-30 seconds per side. This significantly increases the flexibility of the shoulders, which is very beneficial in falls when you land on your shoulder.

3. Upper arms and shoulders

One hand is passed under the chin and laid against the opposite shoulder. Push the elbow toward the shoulder with the other hand.

4. Forearms and wrists

Kneel down and place the hands palms down so that the fingers are pointing directly toward the knees. Now move toward your heels to increase the tension in the forearms and wrists. A similar effect can be achieved by hyperextending the wrists with your arms straight and the palm of the hand facing away from the body and the fingertips pointing downward.

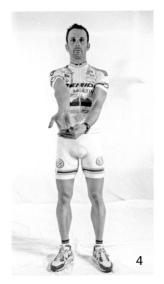
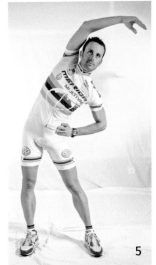
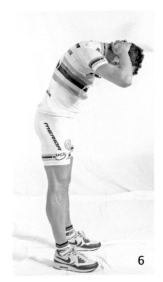

5. Trunk

Stand with the feet roughly shoulder-width apart and bend the upper body to the side, bending one arm over the head with the other resting on the hip.

6. Back and legs

Start by standing up straight. Raise your arms to make yourself very tall, then bring your arms down and start to slowly bend your head to your chest so that first your thoracic spine then your lumbar spine are rounded until finally your upper body is hanging down quite relaxed. Keep your legs straight with your hands almost touching the feet. Then, equally slowly, straighten back up until you are tall again. In this exercise, like the others, make sure that you are relaxed and switched off from outside distractions when you perform it. This is easier to achieve with your eyes closed.

An extremely relaxing exercise for the back is hanging. This involves hanging from one or both arms from a bar or branch, and hang for as long as you are able to hold the position.

7. Hips and lower back

Lying on your back, bring one knee to your chest and hold it there, keeping the other leg straight. In order to stretch the hamstrings, the bent leg can be gripped behind the knee and stretched perpendicular to the body.

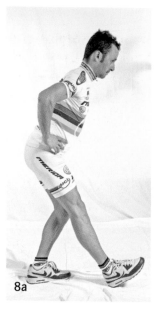
8a

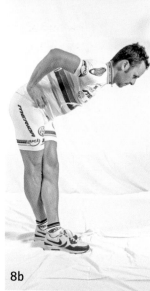
8b

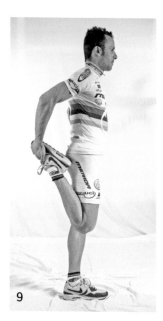
9

8. Hamstrings and calves

a. In the lunge position (feet pointing forward), bend forward, keeping your back straight and your toes pulled back so that you feel a stretch in your calf and hamstrings.

b. With the feet crossed, bend forward keeping your legs straight. Then swap the position of the feet.

9. Quadriceps

Stretching the quads is very important for cyclists. To aid balance, you can rest against a wall when stretching the quadriceps. Grip the instep of the foot with the left hand and raise the foot toward the buttocks. Pull it slowly toward the glutes until you can feel tension in the quads. The hips should be brought slightly forward, making sure that the thighs remain parallel to each other and the upper body is erect. Hold for 20-30 seconds per side.

10. Adductors

Stand in a wide side lunge position with the feet parallel and facing forward. Bend one knee until the stretch can be felt on the inside of the thigh above the knee. This stretch can also be performed in a forward lunge position.

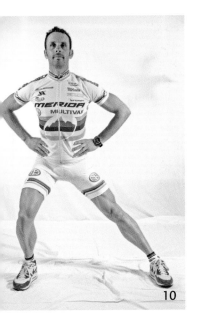
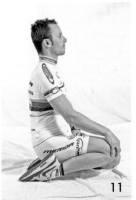
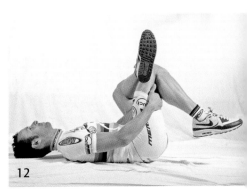

11. Quadriceps and shin muscles

Kneel down with the backs of your thighs and feet on the floor. After about 15 seconds, lift one knee with one hand, stretching the muscles in front of the shin.

12. Glutes

Lie down on your back and stretch out your body. Then raise one leg and place the ankle of the other leg on the knee of the raised leg. Now link hands behind the thigh of the raised leg and pull it slightly toward you, keeping your hips on the floor. If the stretch is not strong enough, push the knee outward slightly.

13. Hamstrings, calves, and back

In the sitting position, place one ankle on the opposite thigh slightly above the knee. Now lean forward, keeping your back straight, possibly with the toes also pulled toward you.

Exercises to strengthen the core muscles

This chapter would not be complete without a few effective exercises for strengthening the core (back, abs, shoulders, lower back) and serve to improve posture. They can easily be integrated into a stretching program.

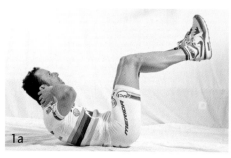
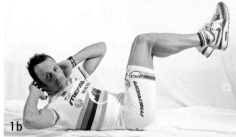

1. Abdominal muscle training

    a. Crunches: Lie on your back. Raise your legs and slowly roll your body up to your legs and down again, starting from the head; 10-20 reps (straight abdominal muscles).

    b. Twisting crunches: In the same starting position, link your hands behind your neck and again roll up slowly, but this time bring your elbow to the opposite knee; 10-20 reps (oblique abdominal muscles).

2. Back muscle training

Lie on your stomach with legs extended behind you. Look at the floor and raise your legs slightly off the floor. Now perform slow, sweeping pull-up movements. Bring the arms back close past the body and then quickly move them forward again and repeat; 15-30 reps.

3. Push-ups

When performed correctly, the push-up is an excellent exercise both for the back and abs and for the arms and shoulders. It is important to maintain good body tension and to keep the body straight. Different variations with narrow and wide arm positions; fast, slow, or markedly high reps are possible. The number of reps is totally dependent on the ability of the individual. Ideally, three sets of predetermined reps should be performed.

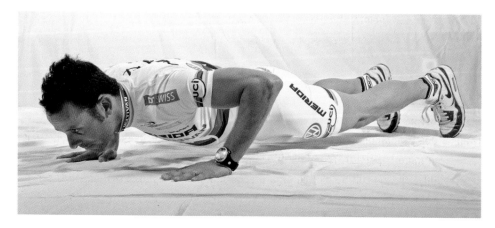

3.10 Training Diary

Recording training data in a diary is referred to by sports scientists as training documentation. These valuable entries can provide the coach and also the cyclist with conclusions relating to training structure, errors to be avoided, and positive aspects to be repeated.

For the recreational cyclist whose main aim is exercise but not achieving peak form, it is sufficient to enter his training mileage combined with a few other pieces of information such as course, weight, resting pulse rate, or weather in a pocket diary, which will give him a clear summary in the form of an end-of-year review.

At high performance level, though, this type of documentation is not sufficient, as considerably more information is required. Measuring daily resting heart rate, weight, training zones breakdown, and physical injuries are just a few points that need to be ordered in an easily comprehensible format. A tried and tested way of doing this is with specially printed training diary sheets that can easily be filed in a folder. This provides all the important training data and race results at a glance. Two sheets are required per month (delete all irrelevant data rows). All sporting activity is entered on the sheets, not just cycling (see table 3.5).

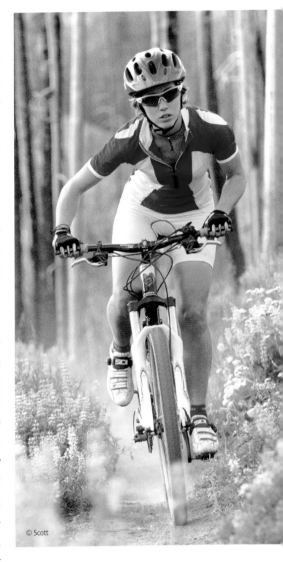

© Scott

Data analysis

Training documentation is more than just collecting data. The evaluation, or training analysis, is even more important. There are different ways of doing this: To start with, the weekly and monthly mileage can be plotted on a graph. In another step, race performances can be added to the graph, from which valuable conclusions can be drawn for the following year.

In addition, the results can be combined with resting pulse rates, the results of performance testing, and any illnesses. A very complex graph can be created from all these values.

At high performance level, distinctions are also made between the different training zones, thus complicating matters further. For the purposes of representation, other time periods than the calendar or training year can be selected, such as the specific preparation for a race or a multi-year overview. These very laborious procedures become important from the junior category onward.

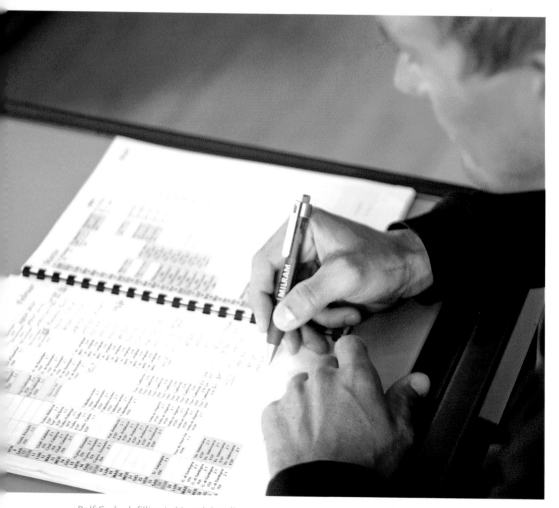

Ralf Grabsch filling in his training diary

Table. 3.5: Training diary

Cycling training diary		Name:				Month:			Category:	
Date	Training distance/race location/other training	Type of training Type of race	No. of riders	Daily mileage	Duration	Monthly mileage	Weight	Resting pulse rate	Comments	
1./16.										
2./17.										
3./18.										
4./19.										
5./20.										
6./21.										
7./22.										
8./23.										
9./24										
10./25.										
11./26.										
12./27.										
13./28.										
14./29.										
15./30.										
31.										

Training sessions on bike:
Other training

Training hours:
(total/bike/other):

Race mileage:
(Month)

Monthly mileage:

Yearly mileage:
Carry foreward:

Before this, only the basic aspects of analysis without graphic display were sufficient. Unfortunately, many cyclists do not keep a training diary let alone analyze it, or the important data wind up in the waste basket at the end of the season and are lost. This is why cyclists should get used to keeping a simple training diary from an early age.

Training plans

Both the coach who prepares training plans for his cyclists and cyclists who prepare their own plans need clear plans that allow them to later monitor their training according to the data entered. The blank training plan provided contains in the top row the required volumes and types of training and in the bottom rows the training that is actually performed, thus enabling a direct comparison of set and actual training. Younger cyclists in particular may be tempted to exaggerate the data in order to look more impressive, even though very little or no training has been done. However, it usually is enough to explain that in this way they are only cheating themselves. If the coach–cyclist relationship is relaxed and friendly, no problems of this nature should arise anyway.

Table 3.6: Training plan template

Week:				Name:	
Day	Date	Mile-age	Content training zones	Extra diet, exercises	Mileage ridden content
Mon.					
Tues.					
Wed.					
Thur.					
Fri.					
Sat.					
Sun.					

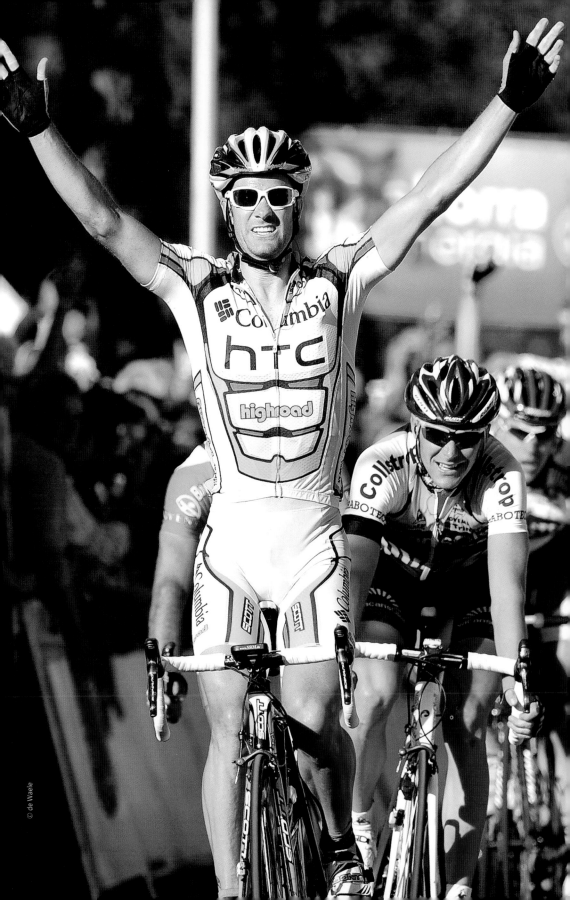

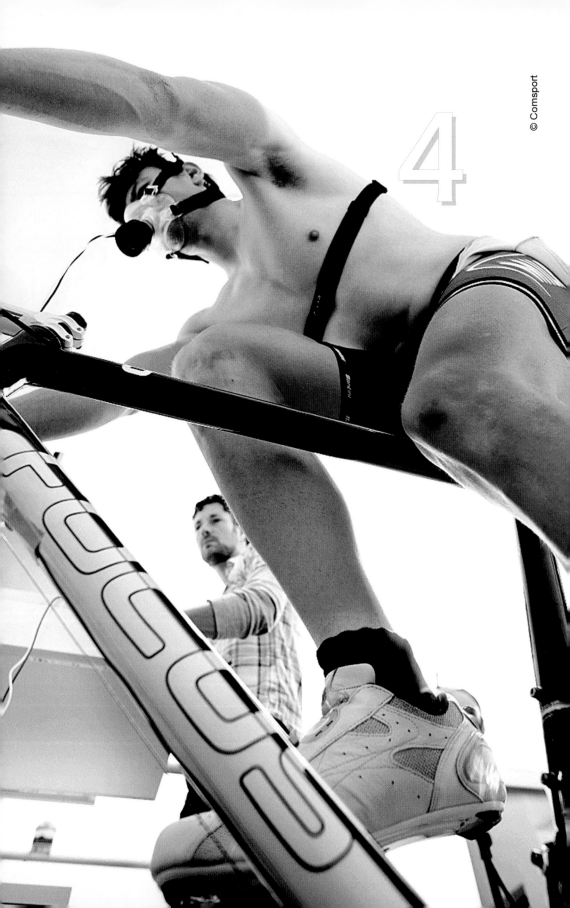

4

4   Performance Diagnostics and Testing

4.1   Lab Tests

Regular performance tests as a means of analyzing performance levels and also managing training have been an integral part of high-performance cycling since the 1970s. Four to six tests are performed annually, at the start and in the middle of the preparation phase and at the start and middle of the racing phase. Performance testing is used in preparation for peak performances in order to identify and correct any weak points in good time.

Too much importance should not be given to the result of a performance test, as peak performances can also be achieved without expensive tests just by means of correct training and experience. Test results may also be influenced by a number of factors that could lead to completely incorrect conclusions about training planning, particularly if the coach or diagnostician lack experience in interpreting results. A single test does not reveal enough information to inform training, so regular testing is required to be able to benefit fully from the process.

The purpose of lab performance tests is to monitor training planning to enable optimal training structuring, because optimized sequencing of planned training and rest are essential for best possible development. Control parameters are power and heart rate, and in track or time-trial training, lactate concentration, not cycling speed.

Stage test

The stage test on a bicycle ergometer suits cyclists as they are familiar with the pedaling action. A bicycle ergometer test would be less suitable for a runner, as the pedaling action on the bike would not allow him to perform to the best of his ability. A treadmill test would be more appropriate for runners, but not for cyclists. The bicycle ergometer must be set up exactly like the cyclist's own racing bike, and he should also use his own pedals and shoes in order to minimize disruptions to the motion sequence.

The exercise intensity is gradually increased in stages, and the cyclist exercises to the point where he is forced to drop out due to exhaustion. Depending on the test protocol and purpose, the stages last between one and six minutes with load increases of 20-50 W per stage.

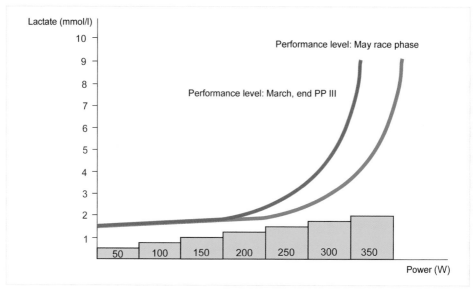

Fig. 4.1: Performance improvement during a training period is measured using two lactate performance curves.

Longer stages of five to six minutes allow the metabolism to adapt and plateau at what is referred to as *steady state*. Shorter stages with high power increases mean that when the results are analyzed, there are excessively high settings for the training intensities due to delayed lactate distribution. The training goal would therefore be missed, unless the results are corrected with a test-specific factor.

New test procedures use very short ramp tests with high power increases in very short stages to study lactate production speeds and interpret them with the aid of complex calculation models.

Standard conditions

The tests must be carried out under standardized conditions, because the type of diet, previous day's training, lactate analysis method, and even air temperature and humidity all have an influence on the test result. To ensure that all tests can be compared with each other, all the tests within a training year must be performed using the same method with identical stage lengths and loading increases. During the test, different measurements can be taken to determine physiological and biomechanical values such as heart rate, electrocardiogram (ECG), cadence, power, ventilatory parameters (oxygen uptake, CO_2 discharge, respiratory minute volume), and lactate, glucose, urea, and creatine kinase concentration.

Spiroergometry, measuring oxygen uptake, is not cheap and drives up the cost of a test. However, determining the ventilatory parameter is advisable and should be carried out if at all possible.

It is not necessary to go into further detail about conducting a stage test in the context of this introduction, as these tests cannot be self-administered anyway. The most important data, which must ultimately be compared with each other, are power, heart rate, and the associated lactate values. If these are represented in graphic form, the lactate performance curve is obtained, which is used to calculate the aerobic and anaerobic thresholds.

Thresholds

For endurance-trained cyclists, the *aerobic* threshold is around 2 mmol lactate/l blood, and the *anaerobic* threshold is around 4 mmol/l, although sports science views differ greatly on this.

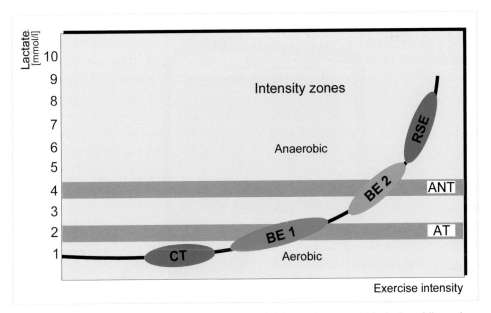

Fig. 4.2: Threshold model and intensity zones. The thresholds are shown as thick shadowed lines whose width corresponds to the possible range of the figures. The intensity zones are represented schematically. AT = aerobic threshold, ANT = anaerobic threshold

When analyzing a curve, you start from a certain lactate value that is related to the corresponding heart rate. So if, for example, the aerobic threshold (lactate 2) is around 150 bpm, then in basic training 1, you should not significantly exceed a heart rate of 150 bpm. The same can also be done for the other training zones, although this does not always lead to a correct differentiation.

It is not possible to give a description for the interpretation of lactate performance curves at this point, because there is no definitive interpretation model. All models have inaccuracies, and, at the end of the day, a performance diagnostician settles on a model that he believes in. If you do not constantly change diagnosticians, you can obtain useable results despite this vague approach.

Performance development

Performance improvement or, more generally performance development, can be traced back accurately using several lactate performance curves. In preventive and rehabilitative therapeutic cycling, lab diagnostics have a very important function; they enable the physician to accurately diagnose performance capacity and the physiotherapist to set the correct training dosage.

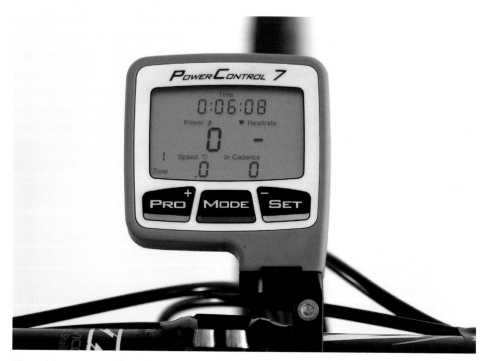

The mobile power meter (SRM) has revolutionized cycling training.

Although in this case the lactate value is usually not calculated, but more importance is attached to the ECG and blood pressure. Once factors that influence the test results have been eliminated, lab diagnostics are the most accurate method for establishing the training zones. This is also the only way of ascertaining and quantifying maximal performance capacity.

Sports science and sports medicine institutes in universities have now tested so many athletes (cyclists) that, based on the data obtained, it is possible to give really accurate principles for setting training zones, which are sufficient for many cyclists. However, there are still inaccuracies as already mentioned.

In general, the higher the performance level, the more crucial a performance diagnostic test is to set the cyclist's training zones, because the margin for error between effective and ineffective training becomes smaller and smaller.

Other lab tests

In the context of the complex cycling-specific performance diagnostic test, not only can the overall performance on the bike be measured, but individual components of this overall performance can be measured with specific tests. Some of these possible tests are: maximal pedaling power, maximal cadence, anaerobic capacity, pulling power as a function of cadence, and pedal power under different loads.

4.2   Field Tests

Prior to the description of simple performance tests in the next section, the field test should be presented as a compromise between the pure lab diagnostics and the very simple time trial test. The field test is a stage test (i.e., increasing loading stages) that is not conducted in a lab under standardized and idealized conditions, but performed in the field (i.e., with your own bike on the road, in the forest, or on the track). The advantage of this test is that it is very practical-oriented; however there are greater potential sources of error. Due to differing external factors (e.g., wind, course, temperature, equipment, tire pressure), it is very hard to compare several tests by the same athlete or simultaneous test by different athletes. If possible, the field test can be conducted on a cycle race track (always the same lap length, wind can be calculated, easy to perform) by road cyclists on a road bike.

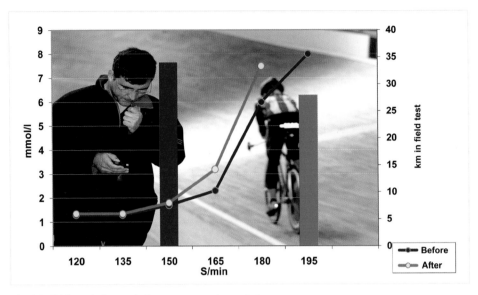

Fig. 4.3: Field test before and after a stage race in a velodrome

Implementation

In the field test, normally only two or three parameters are determined, such as the heart rate and the lactate value as a function of speed. The intensity during the test is either controlled by speed or heart rate, with stage lengths of 2-6 km.

Longer stages are more suitable for very well-trained cyclists to determine the lower training intensities than the short stages (less than 1 km) that are sometimes recommended. For example, start with a speed of 28 km/h that is increased every 2.5 km (for a 250 m track = 10 laps) by 2 km/h.

During the test, the heart rate is shown on the heart rate monitor, and the lactate values are measured after each stage. It is the cyclist's responsibility to stick as closely as possible to the speed or heart rate targets with the aid of his bike computer or heart rate monitor.

In field tests it can be difficult to choose the correct gear ratio to enable the cadence in all stages to remain at a constant 80-100 revs per minute, hence the need for a cadence meter. This means low gear ratios for lower speeds and high gear ratios for high speeds, and it is not easy to adapt them to the exact velocity or heart rate required.

It is even more accurate to structure the stages according to heart rate. This allows you to compare tests taken on different days under differing external conditions (e.g., wind factor). Start at the first stage with 115 bpm, and then increase by 15 bpm for each stage until exhaustion. Speed and lactate are also calculated.

Analysis

To start, plot a graph with the lactate concentration on the left y-axis and the heart rate on the right y-axis. On the x-axis enter the speed (calculate for every stage). Now the individual data pairs are populated to create two data rows: the lactate–speed data row and the heart rate–speed data row. Two curves are formed by connecting the points on a data row.

Interpret the curve by relating a specific lactate value to the corresponding heart rate on the other curve, which might mean that the aerobic threshold lies at a heart rate of 130 bpm, for example. This means that in basic training 1, the heart rate of 130 bpm should not be exceeded.

The aerobic threshold corresponds to the lowest measurement in the lactate–speed curve, provided that it was measured accurately. The anaerobic threshold is calculated by adding 1.5 mmol/l lactate to the aerobic threshold figure. The other training zones are calculated using the lactate values provided in the respective illustrations.

At the end of the day, if you are interested enough and are able to organize it, you should test out this method so that you can form your own opinion.

4.3   Time Trial Tests

As well as lab diagnostics and stage tests, simple performance tests can be conducted individually and inexpensively. These tests should be done as time trials and can be carried out during the preparation and racing phases. They should be done at the end of each training cycle so that training planned for subsequent cycles can be modified if necessary.

A performance test is useful for documenting performance development of newcomers to cycling, particularly for young cyclists. But it can also be used for more experienced cyclists. This kind of performance test is recommended not just for racing cyclists but also for cycling tourists. In order for the results of the performance test to give objective information, the time trial tests must be conducted under similar weather conditions (e.g., same wind factor). The time trials provide the coach with information about the effectiveness of the cyclist's training and are also very motivating for the newcomer to cycling. The newcomer makes big leaps in performance at the start of the training process in the first year, and these are clearly reflected in the performance test.

The first time trials should take place at the start of the preparation phase at the start of the first training cycle. In order to avoid overuse symptoms of the musculoskeletal system, a good

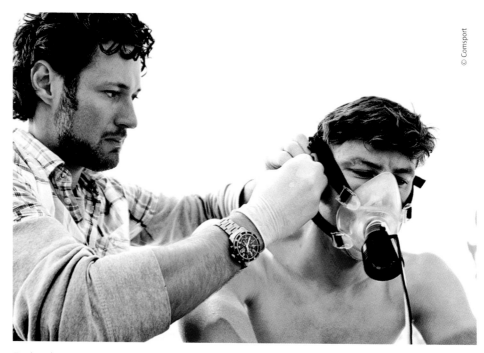

During the stage test, samples of capillary blood are taken from the cyclist's earlobe

pre-test warm-up is essential (at least 30 min), and very heavy gears, which the muscles cannot cope with, should be avoided to maintain a smooth pedaling action. However, if you absolutely do not want to use high gears at the start of the preparation phase, you can do the first three to four tests just with the small chainwheel with a gear ratio of 42 x 16-14, which requires a very high cadence.

It is not sufficient to perform the test just once with a low gear ratio in order to ensure tests are comparable. Only when you have sufficient mileage under your belt can the gear ratio be feely chosen, but it should not exceed the appropriate gear ratio for the category concerned.

Time-trial course

For the performance test, a quiet course with no dangerous curves or descents is required. A circuit has organizational advantages over a straight course. Riding several circuits reveals split times. The course should be between 5 and 15 km long, but for younger teenage cyclists it should not exceed 10 km and for juniors and amateurs it can be up to 20 km. Once a suitable course has been found, it should be put down in writing along with a table in which all times are noted. After several years of training, this also helps track performance development. A coach can also glean valuable comparison values from it, which facilitate the grading of new cyclists.

Several starters

With a starting sequence of 1 minute, when stopping the time with only one stopwatch from the second starter the difference in start time to the first starter must be subtracted. Staggered starts every 1 minute have been proved to be successful.

In the comments column, you can note whether the cyclist had problems with his bike, for example. The how you feel column should be completed before the time trial with marks from 1-10 (1 = very bad, 10 – excellent).

It is advisable to set up two different time-trial courses:

    a. one flat or slightly undulating one
    b. one mountain course in order to assess climbing performance (length 2-5 km)

Table 4.1: Time trial template

Performance test: Time trial _____ Date: _____				
Course: _____				
Weather conditions: _____				
Number of participants: _____				
Starter: (age group)	Time:	Average speed	Comments:	Subjective impession (1-10):
1.				
2. - 1 min:				
3. - 2 min:				
4. - 3 min:				
5. - 4 min:				
6. - 5 min:				
7. - 6 min:				
8. - 7 min:				
9. - 8 min:				
10. - 9 min:				

Timing of performance checks

From the start of the training year to the start of the racing season, there is no point in situating the performance check within a microcycle (week); however, it can be used instead of a race at the weekend. However, if the season has begun, a suitable weekday should be chosen for the test. As Mondays are rest days and Fridays are pre-race days, they can't be used. Tuesdays are usually used for strength and sprint training, so this means that only Wednesdays and Thursdays are possible. You should choose the day when the time trial fits best into the training plan. If there is no race at the weekend, the time trial can take place on Saturday or Sunday, as a kind of race substitute. The training stimulus of a 10- to 30-minute time trial in the long-term endurance I category should not be underestimated as it is places very high demands on the aerobic and anaerobic capacity.

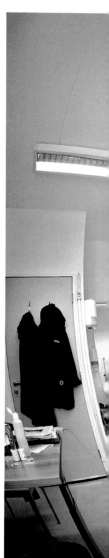

Execution

Warm up thoroughly for 30 minutes before the time trial and follow it with another basic endurance workout. Time trial tests are best done in the training group, because the presence of training partners increases motivation and ambition. Time trails are particularly beneficial for younger cyclists because they are occasions when they can really ride flat out when previously they may have avoided such exertions.

Feeling for pace

When carried out regularly, one benefit of time trials is that they enable cyclists to develop a good feeling for pace so that they can better assess their own endurance performance capacity. Coaches should normally let weaker riders start in front of stronger ones, but, and this is particularly true for younger cyclists, this ranking should be changed in order to prevent frustration and disappointment. It is therefore possible to start two or three equally strong cyclists one after the other and then to leave a slightly greater time gap. The starting order can be set exactly like this. A time gap of one minute has proved to be successful. The timekeeper, usually the coach, remains at the start/finish and notes down the exact starting order and possibly also the split times (see template).

Analysis

Using the times obtained during the season, a meaningful season performance profile can be constructed and can be related to race results or training records (see training documentation).

The times and possibly the split times can also be represented in graph form.

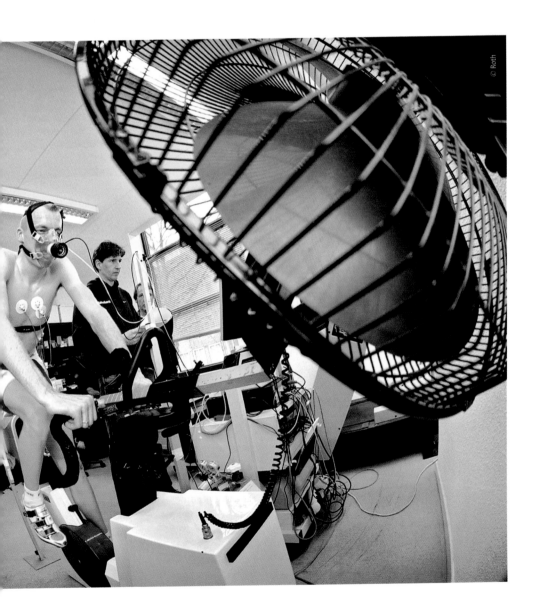

© Roth

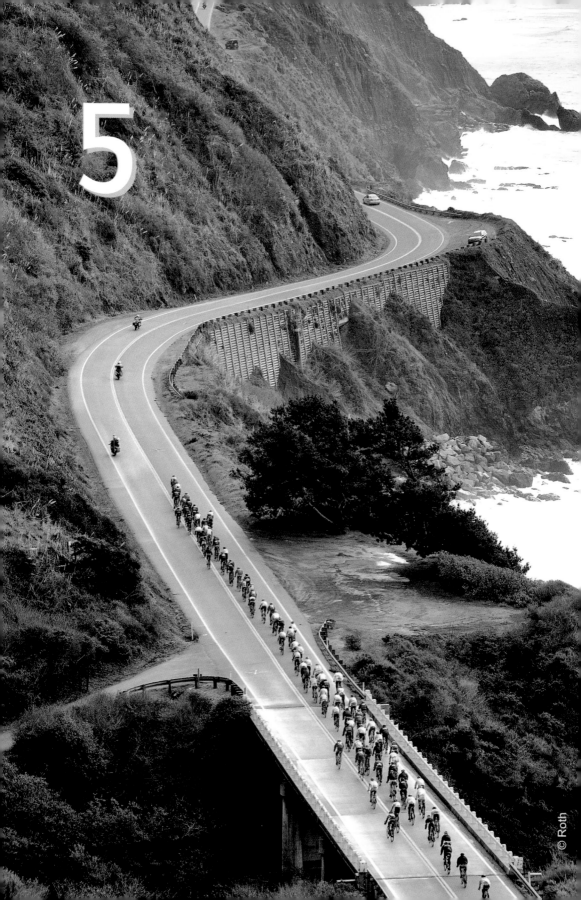

5

© Roth

5   Nutrition

Training volumes and intensities at elite level in endurance sports have increased to previously unimagined levels in recent years. For an increasing number of cyclists, nutrition offers a huge potential for optimization. But by eating well, grass-roots cyclists can also improve their performance, get healthier, and improve their quality of life. Compared to sedentary individuals, very large amounts of food are required and metabolized. Elite athletes should therefore be extremely careful that the food they eat is as high-quality and unprocessed as possible.

In cycling history, athletes, coaches, and managers have always been on the lookout for "miracle" foods or nutritional supplements that will give them an advantage over their opponents. In no other sport are there as many nutrition myths as in cycling. This chapter explains what nutrition is really about and how you can easily eat a sports-appropriate diet.

5.1   Foundations of Nutrition for Endurance Sports

Functions of food:
- Energy supply (for physical activity and vital functions)
- Build-up and maintenance of the body (cells, tissue)
- Regulation of the metabolic processes and health protection (in order to reduce the negative effects of the environment and high-performance sport on the body as much as possible)

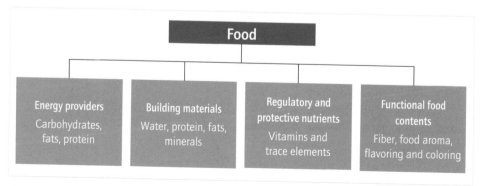

Fig. 5.1: Food groups in sports nutrition

There are four main food groups

1. Energy providers (fuels)

Energy providers are carbohydrates (starch, sugar) and **fats** (lipids). If long endurance feats are performed without adequate carbohydrates, **proteins** are then used for energy production. For example, long distance runners (> 300 km) obtain approximately 10-15% of their energy from proteins. Even the immune proteins in the blood (globulin, albumen) are used, which is the reason for cyclists' increased susceptibility to infection during and after stage races.

Alcohol, with 7 kcal/g, is also considered an energy provider, which often accounts for an unfortunately high proportion of the total amount of energy.

2. Building substances

Proteins are the building blocks of the body; they are involved in the construction of muscles, tendons, ligaments, and cartilage. An important building substance in the body is water, which composes 60% of the human body. Minerals are also building substances. Fats, too, are necessary for the construction of cell membranes and the insulation of nerve cell extensions.

3. Regulatory and protective agents

Vitamins, minerals, and **trace elements** belong to this group. Water also belongs to this group, because it is responsible for heat regulation.

4. Function-supporting nutritional substances

These include **fiber,** as it stimulates the digestion and heightens the feeling of satiety. Our enjoyment of food is greatly dependent on **aromas, flavorings,** and **colorings,** for what good are delicious-looking meals if they didn't taste and smell nice too?

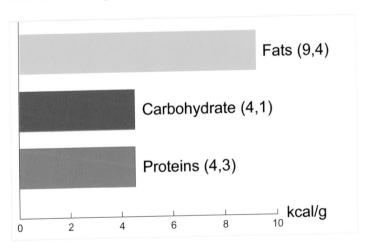

Fig. 5.2: Calorific value of nutrients

Carbohydrates

Carbohydrates play a key role in sports nutrition. They ensure energy supply during heavy training or racing, are easy to digest, and in most cases are also healthy. They have two main advantages: They are both an oxygen-efficient (per liter of oxygen consumed, they provide over 10% more energy than fats) and fast source of energy. In our food, two-thirds of the energy supplied by carbohydrates should be in the form of complex carbohydrates (polysaccharides): over sucrose (household sugar), lactose (milk sugar) and maltose (malt sugar), and starches. Their molecules consist of at least two simple sugars; starch molecules are even constructed of up to 1,000 connected glucose molecules. The simple sugars (monosaccharides) should account for at least one-third, including glucose (dextrose), fructose (fruit sugar), and galactose. Our diet consists of approximately 35-60% carbs, compared to just 40% in the general population in the year 2000, which is too low for athletes. The amount of carbs in the total calorie intake should be at least 60%.

High-carb foods

High-carb foods are pasta, rice, bread, whole grain products, potatoes, honey, marmalade, and fruit. Since the complex carbs (multiple sugars) must be broken down into monosaccharides before they can enter the bloodstream, it is obvious that it is best to consume monosaccharides such as grape or fruit sugar for faster digestion. This method has two snags, though:

1. A fast blood sugar spike caused by the simple sugars (fast absorption) follows an equally fast drop in blood sugar level (an insulin release causes the sugar to be deposited very quickly in the cells), leading to a deterioration in performance or even drop-out. So, do not consume simple sugars before a tour or a race, but only in the final miles when you feel your performance starting to dip and want to maintain it.

2. Simple sugars consist of more molecules per amount of energy than multiple sugars; their osmotic concentration is therefore higher. As the stomach establishes the digestion time of foods based on their concentration; less concentrated foods (e.g., multiple sugars like dextrine) pass through the stomach more quickly and can be absorbed into the blood in the small intestine after being broken down.

Short or long?

A compromise is therefore required between digestion time (concentration) and fast absorption into the blood (type of carbohydrate). For this reason, prepared energy drinks are composed of a combination of different sugars.

So ideally, complex carbs should be consumed before and during exercise and simple carbs toward the end. In training and during tours, simple sugars should be avoided as much as possible.

The storage form of carbohydrates in the body is called glycogen (see chapter 2.2). Glycogen is another macromolecule composed of many simple sugars (glucose). When the body is active, it draws on the glycogen reserves in the liver and muscles.

Fats

While the amount of fats in the total energy should constitute about 25-30%, most Americans eat much more than this, leading to the problem of unused, excessive energy being stored as fatty deposits. A high-fat diet also increases the risk of health problems (e.g., arterial sclerosis). For these reasons, fat consumption should be reduced.

Triglycerides make up 95% of fats consumed by humans and are used for energy production; about 5% of the fats are phospholipids and cholesterol, which are used as building materials. The triglycerides are split into glycerin and free fatty acids and are absorbed in the small intestine by specialized cells and distributed via the lymph system into the circulation. What is not immediately burned for energy production is remade into triglycerides and stored. If the glycogen reserves are depleted during exercise, the stored fat deposits are remobilized and recruited for energy production. The fats can, however, only burn in the "fire of carbohydrates;" if the carbohydrates are highly depleted, fat burning is also diminished, leading to a drop in performance capacity. Fatty foods prolong the length of time food spends in the stomach and therefore delay the absorption of food. They slow down the replenishment of the glycogen reserves that is so important for recovery after exercise.

Fatty foods

Firstly, there is the group of foods that obviously contain fat such as fatty meat, butter, cream, and fried foods. But there is also a whole range of foods including such delicacies as cakes, candy, ice-cream, sauces, dairy products, and sausages which contain an excessive amount of hidden fat. However, sports nutrition is not just about banning all tasty food, but about choosing intelligently, and by avoiding certain treats, the total fat content of the diet can be significantly reduced.

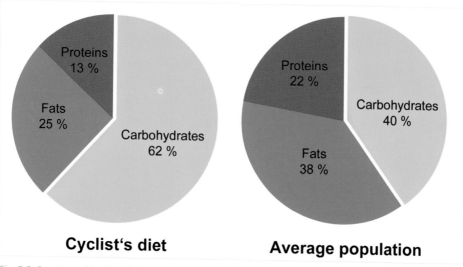

Fig. 5.3: Sports nutrition breakdown

Proteins

Proteins are providers of energy and should account for roughly 10-15% of the total energy requirement. The importance of proteins for performance in endurance sports was long underestimated. This explains the belief that used to be held, and sometimes still is, in cycle racing circles that a daily steak is the basic prerequisite of a sports-appropriate and performance-boosting diet. In fact, the proteins in the cells, in addition to their main function as building and transporting substances, are only minimally involved in energy production.

Proteins consist of chains of different amino acids. There are 22 different known amino acids of which humans must consume 10 in their diet; we are able to synthesize the rest ourselves. In the stomach and small intestine, the proteins are split by enzymes and absorbed as amino acids into the blood. If the specific amino acid requirement in a cell is met, the amino acids are converted into fat and glycogen and also used for energy production. For the endurance athlete, the recommended protein requirement is 1.2-1.5 g per kg bodyweight. An additional protein intake in the form of powders is not necessary. If more protein is consumed, this in no way means that more muscle mass will be built. Instead, the surplus amount is burned up as third-choice fuel and eliminated again as urine, which puts too much stress on the kidneys. You must drink a lot to prevent dehydration in the case of high protein consumption. The other part of the excess protein calories is stored as fat. This makes it clear that the important thing is the fat content and amount of high-quality protein in the diet. You should therefore be mindful of the protein to fat ratio.

High-quality protein

Ideal protein sources are fat-free or low-fat dairy products, whole grain cereal products, rice and pasta, as well as almost all types of fish, poultry, and low-fat cuts of beef, pork, and lamb. Legumes and cereal products are also very low fat sources of protein. By increasing consumption of vegetable protein, you lower the amount of fat and increase the amount of fiber, vitamins, and complex carbohydrates you eat. Protein powder supplements are not necessary for mountain biking as long as you have a balanced diet. Amino acid supplementation should only be done under medical supervision and only for therapeutic reasons.

All wrong?

More recent scientific studies put forward the hypothesis that the high-carb diet described previously is incorrect not only for athletes. A high-protein, high-fat, and low–carbohydrate diet allegedly provide a better energy supply for endurance exercise and break down excessive fat deposits, thus enabling the athlete to reach their target weight more easily. While professional cyclists think rather conservatively in this respect, a few top triathletes are already achieving very good performances with a high-fat and high-protein diet. The difference with cycling, though, is in the racing workload. In triathlon the workload is maintained as evenly as possible, while cycling is characterized by alternating workloads with maximal intensity during attacks. It will certainly be very interesting to see how this development plays out, as the sport of cycling has seen many theories come and go in the last 40 years.

Water

Water accounts for roughly 60% of total bodyweight in adults and slightly more in young people and slightly less in the elderly. Almost all metabolic processes require water as a medium, and nothing would work in the body without it. In endurance sports, the body loses a great deal of water through breathing and sweating, and this loss of water (dehydration) means that the metabolic processes can no longer take place at the required pace. The metabolism slows down, leading to a drop in performance.

During intensive physical activity, including cycling, the body can lose 1-2 l of water per hour of activity, depending on weather conditions, clothing, and exercise intensity. During a training ride, the water loss is around 0.5-1 l per hr; in a ride lasting several hours (e.g., 5-hr workout), the water loss is 2.5-5 l. The increasing sweat production caused by dehydration can raise the body temperature, further intensifying the loss of performance.

Of all food deficiencies, the lack of water has the most rapid and serious effect on performance. For this reason it is essential to be well-hydrated before beginning your workout so that

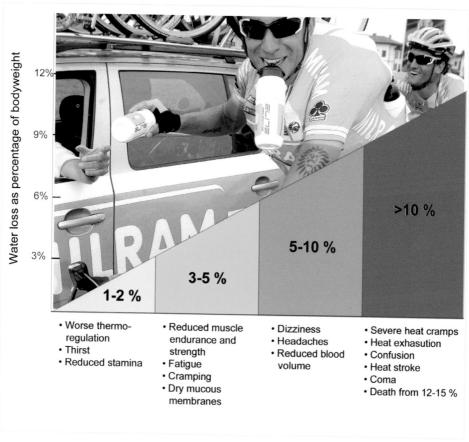

Fig. 5.4: Consequences of exercise-induced water loss

these supplies can be drawn on during exercise. Lost water can be replaced by pure water, as was usual in cycling until recently. Now cyclists mix their own drinks or buy one of the expensive sports drinks promoted by advertising. The advantage of the latter two methods is that as well as replacing the necessary water, they also replace carbohydrates, minerals, and vitamins that are also lost in sweat.

You must remember that minerals are also lost with sweat, not just water.

Hypertonic, isotonic or hypotonic?

The concentration of these drinks is a problem for the manufacturers; on the one hand, they have to be in a form that can be drunk quickly, and on the other they should still contain enough carbohydrates to counteract any decline in performance. For most cyclists, a concentration of 5-8% carbohydrate is most beneficial. So, 5-8 g of carbohydrate is stirred into 100 ml of water (25-40 g in a 500 ml drinking bottle). Higher concentrations (more than 10%) can cause indigestion and stomach problems. However, there are athletes who can even tolerate up to 25% carbohydrate solutions, although this does seem to make little sense from a scientific perspective. The packaging of gels and highly concentrated energy drinks always contain the advice to drink plenty of water afterward.

Personal tolerance levels and the different effect on individuals greatly influence the choice of concentration. Because fruit juice usually has a sugar concentration in excess of 10%, it can be diluted with a good, slightly carbonated magnesium, calcium, and potassium-rich mineral water in the ratio 1:1.

Recent studies show that in endurance workloads lasting up to 3 hours, the mineral deficit can be completely compensated for by the minerals contained in mineral water, and this combined with the carbohydrates contained in the fruit juice is absorbed even more quickly than without the juice into the intestinal tract. However, for normal training rides (90 min), normal mineral water is quite sufficient.

Suitable sports drinks:
- Mineral water (a lot of magnesium, calcium, potassium, and relatively little sodium)
- Fruit juices (especially freshly squeezed)
- Fruit juice spritzers
- Milk, milk shakes (1.5% fat)
- Tea
- Malt beer
- Vegetable juice (ideally without added sugar)

After exercise, fruit juice spritzers are an excellent way of replenishing glycogen reserves due to their relatively high carbohydrate and mineral content.

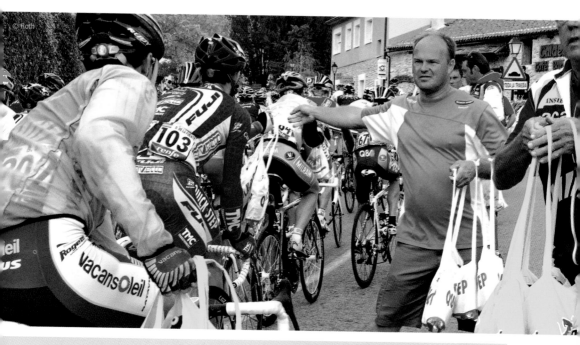

Drinking During Exercise
- Slowly, in small sips
- 150 ml roughly every 15 minutes, not the whole bottle at once
- Never exercise if you are low on fluids or feel thirsty.

The golden rule is to drink regularly during training and racing and definitely before you first feel thirsty. Because once you feel thirsty, the fluid loss is already too great and accounts for about 2% of bodyweight. In high temperatures, take a bottle of ice and drink the thawing cold water, and conversely in the winter, take a thermos of hot tea, which still won't be ice cold even after an hour.

Vitamins, regulatory, and protective substances
Vitamins are organically essential nutrients that influence the metabolism in a great many ways despite only being present in extremely small concentrations. They are not used for fuel by the body and provide no energy. The importance of vitamins for increasing sporting performance capacity is often overestimated, and the actual importance does not justify the indiscriminate use of vitamin products and the addition of vitamins to many processed foods.

However, if you have been diagnosed with a vitamin deficiency, supplements are necessary, but only under medical supervision. Taking vitamins only improves performance if a deficiency existed beforehand. Vitamins are divided into water-soluble and fat-soluble groups:

Fat-soluble vitamins:	A (retinal), D (calciferol), E (tocopherol), K (phyllochinon).
Water-soluble vitamins:	B1 (thiamine), B2 (riboflavin, niacin), B6 (pyridoxin, pantothenic acid, biotin, folic acid), B12 (cobalamin), C (ascorbic acid).

Endurance sports automatically increase vitamin requirements, but this is normally covered by the greater amounts of food eaten, especially if whole grain products are consumed.

Although vitamin supplements probably do not improve performance, at elite level they do protect cyclists from the effects of overtraining. These athletes' bodies are pushed to the extreme, which is rarely the case for normal competitive cyclists, so vitamin supplements can be beneficial. In the case of a reduction in bodyweight, it can happen that the reduced food consumption can lead to a vitamin deficiency, but the deliberate choice of vitamin-rich foods (fruit, vegetables, dairy products) and multivitamin products can cover this in most cases.

Vitamin tablets

Be careful when taking vitamin supplements more than the recommended amount, as negative side effects exist for overdoses of nearly all vitamins, probably also for vitamin C. For this reason, vitamin supplementation must always be discussed with a competent physician. Most relevant for endurance athletes are vitamins B1, B2, E, and C, and these can be supplemented if necessary. Vitamins E and C also have an antioxidative effect (i.e., reduction of cell-destruction by oxidation).

Minerals

Minerals are inorganic elements and compounds, which play a very important role in the human body as building and regulatory substances. They also include the following trace elements: iron, zinc, chromium, selenium, copper, iodine, molybdenum, cobalt, and manganese.

Sodium (Na)

Sodium is essential to maintain the water balance and to activate certain enzymes. It mostly exists in the form of sodium chloride, more widely known as common salt, of which the body contains about 100 g in dissolved form. While a daily sodium intake of 5-7 g is considered adequate, the average consumption in the western world is more than double this. Although common salt is mostly eliminated from the body and exists in high concentrations in sweat, cases of salt, or sodium, deficiency are very rare, because people eat too much salt anyway. Cyclists with a good endurance training background have developed an adaptation mechanism to cope with increased sweating, in which the sweat contains much lower amounts of sodium. The sweat concentrations of magnesium and potassium are unchanged, though.

Magnesium (Mg)

Magnesium is the key mineral in the energy metabolism, as it activates nearly all enzymes, over 300 different ones, involved in it. Unlike sodium but like potassium, it exists almost exclusively within the cells. Sweat contains very large amounts of magnesium; it is several times more concentrated in sweat than in blood and should be replaced by magnesium supplements if necessary. A magnesium deficiency has a whole range of symptoms; headaches, fatigue, and muscle cramps are particularly common. As cyclists should do what they can to prevent this, a high-magnesium diet is recommended. Magnesium-rich (over 120 mg/l) mineral water alone will meet the daily magnesium requirement of 600-800 g per day. But only 35-55% of the magnesium consumed is actually reabsorbed. Magnesium reabsorption is negatively influenced when consumed at the same time as fat, protein, alcohol, calcium, or phosphorus.

Calcium (Ca)

Calcium plays an important role in muscle contraction and in the nervous system, which explains why muscle cramp is one of the most obvious symptoms of a calcium deficiency. Only 1% of the body's calcium exists in a free form, as the vast majority (99%) is stored in the skeleton (about 1,000 g) and can be mobilized to a limited extent if required. Most of our calcium requirement (1.5-2.5 g/day) can be covered by dairy products, which is also the reason why non-dairy eating vegetarians find it very difficult to cover their calcium requirement with their usual diet. Children and pregnant women have a higher calcium requirement than adults due to bone growth.

Potassium (K)

During heavy sweating, the body also loses large amounts of sweat, which, like calcium, has an important function in muscle contraction. As potassium is required for glycogen synthesis, a cyclist should have a high-potassium diet. The daily requirement of potassium is between 3-6 g. Potassium deficiency leads to weak muscle contraction and slower recovery, and in severe cases even heart problems have been observed.

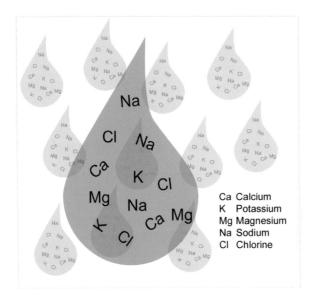

Ca Calcium
K   Potassium
Mg Magnesium
Na Sodium
Cl Chlorine

Phosphorus (P)

Phosphorus exists mainly as a calcium compound in the skeleton. Phosphorus is also an important element for cyclists, because it plays an important role as a building agent in the energy metabolism (formation of ATP). Endurance sport greatly increases the body's phosphorus requirement, which can be covered by an increased sodium intake.

Fig. 5.5: Mineral loss through sweat

Iron (Fe)

Iron is present in the body in a wide range of different compounds and is mainly important for the oxidative metabolism and for oxygen-binding in the red blood pigment (hemoglobin) and muscle pigment (myoglobin). In order to maintain the body's iron levels at 4-5 g, men need a daily supplement of 10 mg of iron, while women need a greater amount (15 g) due to the loss of menstrual blood. The relatively poor iron reabsorption of 10% relative to consumption often results in anemia for female athletes. Anemia, which can only be accurately diagnosed by a blood test, is characterized by reduced physical capacity, fatigue, poor concentration, and sometimes even cardiovascular problems. If anemia is diagnosed, it is essential to treat it. Athletes are generally assumed to have a higher daily iron requirement of up to 25 mg. Vegetarians in particular must be careful to consume enough iron, as the iron in meat is reabsorbed better than that contained in vegetarian food.

Trace elements
Zinc (Zn)

Zinc is the activation agent for over 100 different metabolic enzymes. In order to avoid a zinc deficiency (possible symptoms are inflammatory diseases of the skin and mucous membranes), you should take 15 mg of zinc per day. Fish, meat, dairy, and whole grain products are particularly rich in zinc.

Selenium (Se)

Selenium is also an activator for different enzymes. At only 50-200 micrograms per day, the body requires very tiny amounts (traces) of this still very important element. Evidence is growing that a selenium deficiency can be related to fatal sudden heart attacks in athletes. Selenium is essential for the immune system and certain organs and tissue (liver, muscles, heart, joints); a deficiency affects these structures first. Studies have shown that elite athletes with low selenium levels can increase them and avoid the danger of deficiency symptoms by taking selenium supplements. Supplementation should always be done under medical supervision, as excessive doses of selenium are poisonous. In general, the fact is that science is still in its infancy when it comes to trace elements and their effects. This area of sports nutrition will surely see some interesting discoveries in the future.

Chromiun (Cr)

The element chromium, hitherto only known in the context of chrome-plated metal, is an equally essential trace element, tiny amounts of which influence the carbohydrate metabolism. Too little is still known about this, though, for sport nutrition advice or dosage to be given.

5.2   Basic Training Nutrition

Balanced sports nutrition also reduces the risk of suffering from lifestyle diseases such as arteriosclerosis, high blood pressure, and cancer.

Features of nutrition for endurance athletes:
- High-carbohydrate
- Low-fat
- High-protein
- Varied
- No alcohol or nicotine

How do you eat a high-carbohydrate diet?

Pasta, rice (both mainly as whole grain products), whole grain products (whole grain bread, biscuits, all kinds of muesli), potatoes, legumes (beans, peas), vegetables, and fruit as well as fruit juices are excellent *sources of carbohydrates*, which, unlike refined products, also contain a lot of other valuable nutrients. White sugar or white flour for example contain only empty calories, because they contain no other nutrients such as vitamins, fiber, or minerals in addition to the sugar or starch molecules. The same applies to refined flour. A balanced mixture of whole grain products and traditional conventional products appears to be the best kind of nutrition, as the exclusive consumption of whole grain products is very hard on the digestive system. Make sure food is as natural and unprocessed as possible and avoid ready meals and products, which almost always contain additives (flavor enhancers, coloring, preservatives, emulsifying agents).

What to bear in mind in a low-fat diet:

First, your consumption of visible fats (e.g., oil, butter, margarine, meat fat) must be deliberately reduced, and second, you need to be able to identify and avoid hidden fats. Hidden fats are mainly found in fatty sausage, fatty cheese, eggs, candy, sauces, and fried foods. The aim of a low-fat diet is not the banning of all fat consumption, but the conscious selection of food, including the avoidance of unhealthy and fatty food. It is very important to differentiate between saturated and nonsaturated, high-quality fatty acids, which, like linoleic acid, can reduce cholesterol levels unlike the saturated fatty acids. Fats that are liquid at room temperature are of higher quality than solid ones.

Which foods contain high-quality protein?

Cyclists do not need to eat a steak a day to cover their protein requirements. Meat should just be an accompaniment to the high-carb food on the plate and not vice versa. The aim is to reduce the high proportion of meat protein and to replace it with vegetable proteins such as rice, pasta, rye, legumes, soya, potatoes, and oats. Eating more vegetable protein reduces the amount of fat, increases the amount of fiber, and adds vitamins and complex carbs to the diet. Other healthy sources of energy are low-fat dairy products and fish.

Protein powder supplements are unnecessary for cyclists who have a balanced diet. Specific supplementation with certain amino acids should only be done under medical supervision and should only be done for therapeutic reasons.

In general, an elite athlete's diet should be sparing but high-quality in order to be able to achieve a small weight loss or to maintain racing weight. During periods of high training intensities and frequent races, this should be abandoned. The plain diet is especially important in winter, when training is reduced, to avoid putting on weight.

5.3 Pre-Race Nutrition

Although the following sections use the terms competition or race, they can easily apply to long bike tours or tourist rides during which you would like to perform to the best of your ability. Experimenting with diet should be avoided during races. If you want to test a new product or food, do it in training where any digestive issues have less serious consequences.

Some tips:

- In the days leading up to the race, ensure a high proportion of carbohydrates (65%).
- Can possibly use carbohydrate loading (see next section).
- The evening before the race, eat an easily digestible, high-carbohydrate, low-fat meal (pasta party).
- Ensure sufficient fluid intake (no alcohol).
- The last, solid, high-carbohydrate meal should be eaten no more than 3-4 hours before the race and must be easy to digest.
- Don't eat too much, but drink plenty.

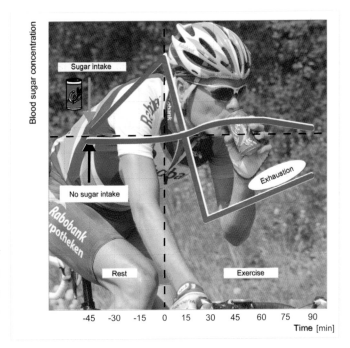

Fig. 5.6: Large amounts of simple sugars consumed shortly before a race lead to undesirable blood sugar fluctuations.

Carbohydrate loading

Carbohydrate loading just means the deliberate filling of the glycogen reserves before a significant load in order to be able to maintain high speeds for as long as possible. Even cyclists whose glycogen reserves are already enlarged compared to other athletes due to their high-carb diet can top off with a bit more. This is done by following a tough, glycogen–reserve-depleting training ride with no food intake with two to three days of reduced training volume and intensity while eating a very high-carbohydrate diet. This has the effect of filling the glycogen reserves, especially in the legs, to a greater extent than before (supercompensation). For a race at the weekend, therefore, Wednesday or Thursday are good days for the exhausting workout.

Before using carbohydrate-loading for an important race, you should first try it out in a few minor races in order to learn how it affects your body.

High glycogen concentrations cause increased water retention in the muscles, which can make the legs feel heavy at the start of the race, but this feeling soon disappears. Carbohydrate loading is only recommended for trained athletes, as no similar supercompensation has been observed in untrained individuals, and large carbohydrate intake could lead to weight gain.

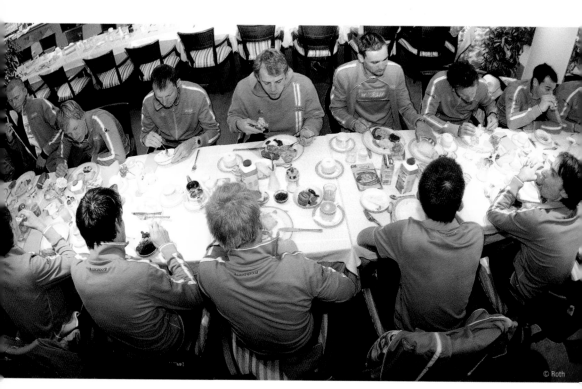

© Roth

Table 5.1: Training and nutrition plan for carbohydrate loading

Training and nutrition plan for carbohydrate loading		
Day	**Training**	**Nutrition**
Thursday 3	Exhausting training depending on age and ability 2-6 hrs BE 1 or 2 with a few tempo sections (RSE), either with the road bike entweder or the MTB, not too much muscular effort	During training: eat as little as possible, drink a lot. Afterward: eat a lot of carbs as soon as possible.
Friday 2	Depending on age and ability, 1-3 hrs BE 1/CT, easy pace, as little muscular effort as possible	High-carb, low-fat food Breakfast: muesli, bread Lunch: pasta, rice, potatoes Dinner: pasta, rice, potatoes
Saturday 1	Depending on age and ability, 1-2 hrs BE 1/CT, easy pace, 1 x 1-4 min BE 2/RSE to test	High-carb, low-fat food Like Friday, but pasta party in the evening = large portion of carbohydrate (not too late!), drink as much water as possible.
Sunday 0	Race	High-carb, easily digestible breakfast, possibly a high-carb lunch, 3-4 hrs before, don't eat too much, no cola.

In the carbohydrate loading described in the table, the exhausting workout is performed on a Thursday, but it can also be done on a Wednesday, thus prolonging the loading phase by a day. This kind of performance diet is sometimes specialized even further by eating an extremely high-fat and high-protein diet before embarking on the carbohydrate loading phase described earlier. Nutrition and specific diets should not become a punishment though; the food should be just as tasty as before. For this reason, carbohydrate loading should only be used in the preparation of really important races.

5.4   Nutrition During the Race

It is only necessary to eat during races lasting longer than 60 minutes. If the race lasts longer than 90 minutes, it is essential to consume carbohydrates in order to avoid a drop in performance. In training, depending on your training state, a small carbohydrate snack is only required after about two hours.

Hitting the wall

In cycling, the state of total exhaustion of the carbohydrate reserves is called bonking or **hitting the wall**. Typical symptoms such as hallucinations of food, dizziness, loss of concentration, disorientation, and significantly reduce performance level can indicate a state that can be very dangerous on a racing bike in traffic. In order to raise the now very low blood sugar level, it is usually sufficient to eat a few sugar lumps or some glucose. Although this does not significantly improve the performance level, you will quickly feel better and will then be able to return

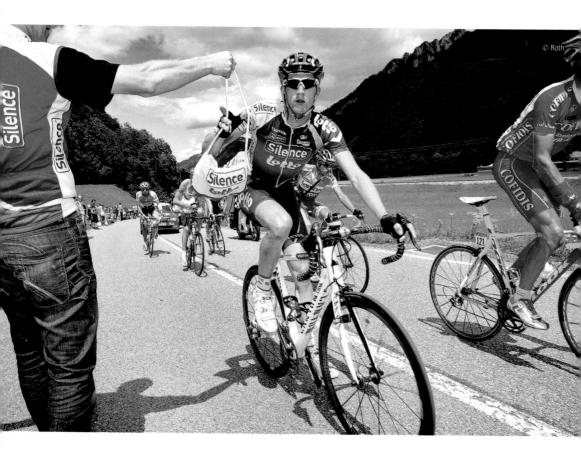

© Roth

home or search for food with a clear head. The wall usually affects cyclists in spring in the first longer training rides in the still-cold, damp air. The consumption of high-carbohydrate snacks (especially muesli bars), fruit (banana, apple, pears, dried fruit), rice cakes, bread (with low-fat spread), cookies, and also energy bars prevents you from hitting the wall and maintains performance levels. These foods are cut into bite-size portions and wrapped in aluminum foil. These foil-wrapped treats are very popular with professional cyclists, as they get tired of only eating energy bars.

A basic rule of sports nutrition is that it must be tasty; this is especially true for food consumed during races.

Fluid intake is covered in the previous section, Water. On longer tours, complex carbs are consumed first; then the simple sugars (glucose) are only consumed near the end of the ride. In order to get an energy boost for the often-decisive final spurt, about 30 minutes before the end, many cyclists drink a little coffee with plenty of sugar or cola.

Eating on the bike requires practice, as many newcomers to cycling often cannot eat while cycling due to stomach problems. The ability to eat while cycling is a detail that is often overlooked, and, particularly during longer tours and stage races, considerable amounts of food must be often consumed on the bike. During the last 15-30 minutes of a race, eating solid food can sometimes cause nausea.

Tear off energy bar wrappers as soon as possible before the start of the race or tour and tuck the bars into your jersey so that they are easy to find during the race. Fruit and bread are wrapped in aluminum foil.

5.5   Post-Race Nutrition

Post-exercise nutrition plays a key role in recovery. The depletion of glycogen stores increases the activity of the enzyme glycogen-synthase, which promotes glycogen formation and storage in the cells. As the concentration of this enzyme is highest two to four hours after exercise but then reverts to the starting level after 24 hours, the cyclist must consume sufficient carbohydrates after racing or training to refill his glycogen stores. If this is not done and exercise is resumed the following day, the stores will be emptied further because they have not been refilled.

So glycogen stores are not only emptied by long, intensive exercise, but also by shorter bouts of exercise on consecutive days without refilling the stores in between.

During the first 24 hours after an exhausting race or training ride, there is no difference between using complex or simple carbohydrates, but after 24 hours, complex carbs significantly increase glycogen synthesis. In addition, complex carbohydrates are more advantageous for health reasons, because they can be absorbed in combination with numerous other nutrients and dietary fiber. After exercise, food like pasta, rice, whole grain products, or fruit should be eaten.

Fluid intake

Make use of the two hours immediately after exercise that are usually characterized by a lack of appetite by consuming high-carbohydrate drinks (fruit juice, not too acidic, and cola) for recovery. Normally, special energy drinks can be avoided, unless you are taking part in a multi-day race or a stage race where you are pushing yourself to the limit and the recovery time is very short. The fluid loss should be replaced gradually and not all at once. Ice-cold drinks should be avoided due to the increased sensitivity of the gastrointestinal tract. Fruit juices (rich in potassium, to enhance glycogen storage) diluted with good-quality mineral water restore the fluid balance and also supply minerals and carbohydrates.

5.6   Weight Problems: Obesity

Energy balance is the concept that is essential to understanding obesity. If an individual consumes a certain amount of calories that he cannot use up, then part of the excess is eliminated and the other larger part is stored in the body in the form of fat. In the long term, this person will put on weight. However, if he eats less than he uses up, he will definitely lose weight, because he is forced to draw on his energy reserves in the form of adipose tissue in order to provide the required energy. The deposits are not depleted as much as may initially be imagined though, because the body gets used to the reduced calorie intake and reduces its basal metabolic rate.

This somewhat simplified view reveals the two decisive factors of the energy balance:

    a. Calorie intake
    b. Exercise-related calorie consumption (the more you move, the more you use)

Effective movement

So this means that to lose weight effectively, it is not sufficient just to reduce your food and calorie consumption; instead, the body needs to burn more calories than it consumes and that can only be done through exercise, ideally the classic endurance sports like cycling (also running and swimming). If the bodyweight is constant for a long period of time, then calorie consumption and use are in equilibrium. However, a constant weight does not mean that you have reached your ideal weight. Only high workloads and therefore high calorie consumption allow cyclists to eat very large amounts of food without putting on weight, and many even lose weight as the season progresses.

The problem in our western society is eating too much of the wrong foods combined with a chronic lack of exercise. If weight needs to be lost, it must be done gradually, as a drastic starvation diet would only harm the body. If you just think how long it took to put on the unwelcome pounds, it should be obvious that a weight loss of 20 lb in 2 weeks, as many diets claim to do, is impossible.

20 kg-7,500 km

Another sample calculation for subcutaneous fat: A male who is 20 kg overweight can ride for about 250 hours with his 20 kg of fat (180,000 calories), with an approximate energy consumption of 12 kcal (at 30 km pace) per minute. This would correspond to a distance of around 7,500 km, just using the body's own fat reserves. This rough, simplified, theoretical example is intended to show how much energy is contained in adipose tissue and how long it takes to get ride of this surplus weight. If you now reduce your calorie intake and gradually do more exercise, the energy balance moves into negative territory and the subcutaneous fat will disappear. A diminished appetite due to hormonal changes caused by high amounts of exercise makes it easier to eat less. Equally important as the two points mentioned is the change in eating habits. Particularly when eating less, you should ensure that your diet is balanced and high-quality.

What sounds so simple in theory is hard to put into practice, as there is also a psychological component involved. Laziness, habit, and greediness often get in the way of successful weight loss.

How to lose weight by training

As fat is the main cause of obesity, training should burn as much fat as possible. Relatively long distances at low intensity and not the famous "training time trials" at 33 km/hr are what is needed. On these short training rides, usually over a fixed route, cyclists try to break their old record every time, so the intensity is too high. This means that the energy requirement is mainly met by the burning of glycogen. So no weight is lost, because after training, low blood sugar levels make eating essential, and often more is eaten than is necessary.

The type of training program is naturally dependent on the cyclist's fitness level. For an average-fit touring cyclist, a training duration of about two to four hours with an average speed of less than 27 km/hr (in summer, on a flat course) is recommended, although this would depend to a great extent on the weather, type of course, and size of the training group. A simple way of ensuring the correct training load is that you should be able to talk comfortably during the entire ride. It is also easy for heart rate monitor users to train in the fat burning zone. The optimal training heart rate is normally about 180 minus age. The 50-year-old would therefore do his endurance training with a heart rate of around 130 bpm. However, individual fitness levels should also be taken into consideration, for if the cyclist is unfit, 130 bpm would already be too high.

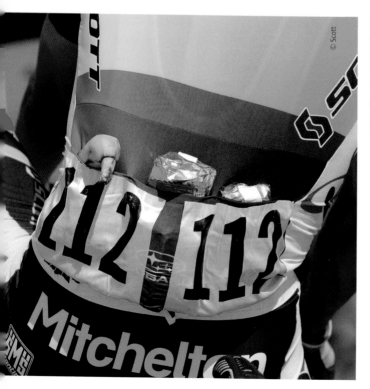

© Scott

If you don't have time for four-hour basic endurance rides, then more intensive, short rides can also achieve the desired results as long as you can restrain your appetite after training.

Food diary

Keeping a food diary is a great help when changing your diet, because it shows all your dietary lapses clearly in black and white. You enter everything you eat during the day, and if you look back the following day you will be amazed at how many different things you eat. Just noting the food for a few weeks makes you much more aware of what you are eating. A simple food diary could look like this:

Date	Time	What?/How much?	Place	Comments

5.7   Weight-Cutting

Normally, the term weight-cutting is only used in combat sports where the athletes starve themselves and avoid water just before competitions to be able to compete in a certain weight category. Fortunately, this is unnecessary in cycling. However, the term can be also be used in this sport. In cycling, though, it does not involve a brief phase a few days before the competition, but a longer process of weight reduction that takes months to complete.

Every racing cyclist is familiar with the connection between form and weight; the better your form, the lower your weight. Here we are talking about racing weight, which is different for everyone depending on their constitution and lies between 2 and 8 kg below your winter weight. In general, your winter weight, when training is cut back, should not deviate significantly from your racing weight.

Weight down, performance up

Often, mountain bikers experience a big performance improvement after losing weight. However, this procedure only really makes sense for elite cyclists, as the already well-trained grassroots cyclist who is at his ideal weight is not so concerned with maximizing his performance and so doesn't need to go to this trouble.

A reduction in bodyweight causes the relative VO_2max to increase, which is the key criterium for performance. The relative VO_2max depends on bodyweight. The athlete's weight drops at constant or even higher absolute performance capacity with the result that he can cycle faster.

Professional cyclists are the athletes with the lowest proportion of adipose tissue; their skin, particularly on their legs, is wafer-thin and is testament to their outstanding and also extreme fitness. The aim should not be to get such thin skin, but just to lose a few more pounds, as even fit amateurs are probably still slightly overweight. Dropping these pounds would enhance their performance. Long training rides in the fat burning zone, especially in the preparation phase, and a light, reduced calorie diet are easy ways of burning off a few pounds.

Your diet should be extremely low-fat, but completely meet your protein requirements in order to prevent muscle protein from being metabolized. Also the carbohydrate supply must be adequate to prevent glycogen depletion.

5.8   The Vegetarian Diet and Cycling

Recent years have seen a boom in vegetarian diets, particularly among endurance athletes, which has brought plenty of food for thought and positive changes to the field of sports nutrition. However, not much has changed yet. There are three different types of vegetarianism:

1.   the vegan, who only eats vegetable products;

2.   the lacto-vegetarian, who also eats dairy products; and

3.   the ovo-lacto-vegetarian, who also eats eggs and egg dishes.

Strict vegetarian or vegan diets should be avoided by elite cyclists; however, a ovo-lacto-vegetarian diet meets all the requirements of a sports diet, as long as the food is high quality (especially the protein intake) and varied.

A high proportion of carbohydrates in the diet is taken for granted. However, meeting iron requirements is more difficult for all three types of vegetarian diet, as meat contains relatively high amounts of iron and this animal iron is more easily reabsorbed than vegetable iron. In any case, iron deficiencies are more commonly found in athletes, especially female, than in non-athletes.

5.9   Alcohol

Alcohol has always been a controversial issue as far as sports nutrition is concerned. "A couple of beers won't do any harm" or "A glass of wine a day is healthy!" are remarks that are often heard. Although they may contain a grain of truth, in grass-roots and elite sport they are only partly correct. There is no scientific evidence of the positive physiological influence of alcohol.

A few facts: 2 l of beer contains 400-450 kcal depending on the type, while malt liquor contains up to 600 kcal (1 g alcohol = 7 kcal). These are not negligible quantities of energy and often the pointer on the scales reveals which lead to an excessive calorie intake and thereby tip the energy balance into positive territory (weight gain). What's more, the consumption of alcohol also stimulates the appetite. For the elite cyclist who trains extremely hard, this is not a problem, but for the grass-roots cyclist, it might lead to a beer gut. In addition, beer also encourages tissue dehydration, as it hardly contains any salt. The result of beer consumption after training or racing is impaired rehydration.

When drunk the evening before a race (morning after thirst), beer disturbs the water balance, and the athlete dehydrates more quickly and his performance deteriorates. Any form of alcohol consumption also fundamentally increases the elimination of magnesium in the urine, thus impairing glycogen synthesis in the recovery phase. In view of all these disadvantages, the consumption of alcohol should be avoided at the very least before and after a race and only enjoyed in extreme moderation at other times.

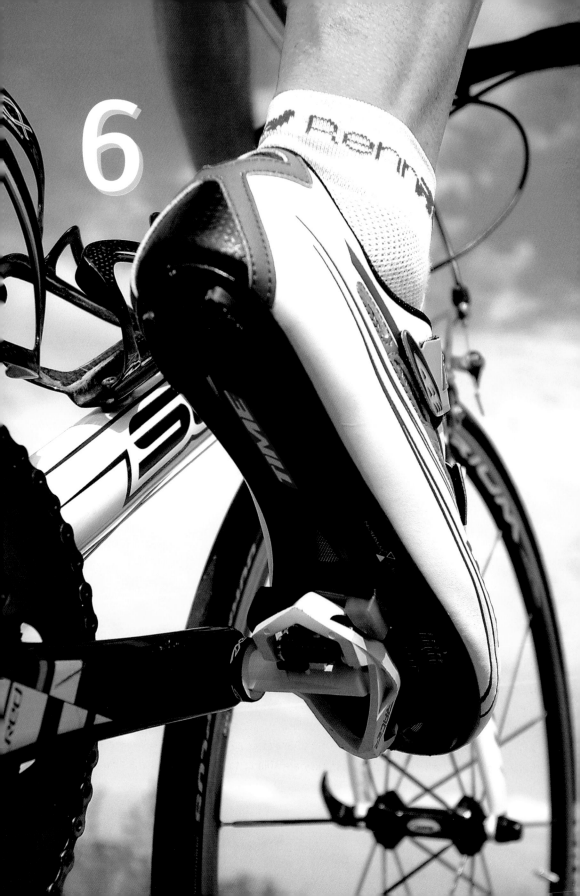

6

6   Medical Aspects of Cycling

6.1   Sports Injuries and Overuse Damage

Excluding traffic accidents, cycling is one of the safest sports. Despite this comparatively low injury rate, the occasional very serious injuries may be sustained in falls and accidents. In general, cycling has an incontestably healthy effect on the human body. In this chapter, the different cycling-specific complaints are explained and tips are given to determine their cause.

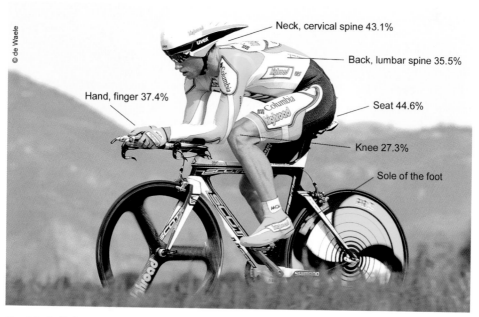

Fig. 6.1: Cyclist's aches and pains (Source: Project Wellcom, DSHS Cologne)

Sports injuries

On many occasions, injuries contracted while cycling do not require medical attention because they are not serious. Most injuries are caused by defective tires or other equipment defects and collisions with other road users. The majority involve grazes, bruises, and slight sprains. An American study (Bohlmann, 1981) shows that 98% of injured cyclists are back in the saddle training after only a week. At the latest, they are able to take part in races again within a month.

Overuse injuries and sports injuries

Overuse injuries occur when the effects of repeated actions exceed the tolerance limits of certain anatomical structures. These injuries usually affect the musculoskeletal system (muscles, tendons, bones, ligaments and joints).

Overuse injuries to the joints and tendons are especially common if build-up training is attacked too hard and too intensively. The muscles, as well-vascularized tissue, react much more quickly to training stimuli and show a more functional adaptation than only poorly vascularized tissue like cartilage, ligaments and tendons. The muscles, therefore, soon become too strong for the weakly vascularized tissue, leading to injuries. The vascular deficiency (bradytrophy) of this tissue is also the reason why, once injuries have occurred, they take a long time to heal. Slow healing is also due to the extremely slow metabolism in tendons, ligaments, and cartilage.

The tolerance limit for mechanical stimulation is determined by many factors and very different from one individual to another, although a sensible and gradual training structure would seem to play an important role. Cyclists seem to tolerate overuse injuries and associated pain for much longer than comparatively minor injuries. This is, of course, related to cyclists' ability to put up with sustained exercise-related pain.

Another piece of American research (Vetter, 1985) showed that it takes racing cyclists an average of 4.8 months from the first signs of overuse injury to consultation with medical specialists. It is probably that ignoring the pain in this way made the injuries even worse and made healing more difficult and slow-going. Overuse injuries often arise due to an incorrectly set-up bike or defective pedals or cranks.

The following sections deal with both typical cycling injuries and also general sports injuries. Using the knee as an example, it is made clear how complex and hard it can be to pin down the cause of overuse injuries.

6.2 Orthopedic Problems

The majority of medical problems in cycling are orthopedic ones (i.e., they affect the structures of the musculoskeletal system). The sitting position on the bike, in which the bodyweight is borne by the racing bike, means that the forces acting on the musculoskeletal system are really low and even with no peak loads like in running. There are many examples of athletes, even at the very highest levels, who have had to change sports due to joint problems and have chosen cycling due to its low-impact nature. If cyclists do suffer from joint pains, in most cases they can be traced back to injuries or overuse not caused by cycling. The legs are a perfect example to help better understand injuries and overuse damage.

a) Hips

Hip joint problems are extremely rare in cycling, as there is very little stress on the hips, unlike in running. Pains that radiate into the hips often originate from a slipped disc or other trapped nerve. When they do happen, hip pains are often the result of an incorrect sitting position or pedaling action.

b) Knee

The knees suffer most in cycling, because they must tolerate the greatest pushing and pulling forces and are exposed to the cold airstream. Compared to runners, cyclists have fewer knee problems. Degenerative changes (arthritis) are much less common than in runners. Unlike in running, the knees are not required to absorb shock, and they are not vulnerable to sprains and bruising as they are in many ball games.

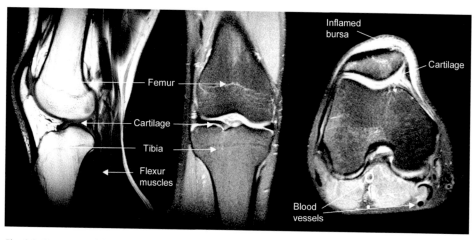

Fig. 6.2: Structures of the knee joint (MRI scan)

Falls onto the knees are the greatest danger for knees in cycling. Ligament injuries caused by the rotation of the lower leg against the upper leg only occur in falls when the feet get stuck in the pedals. In falls onto the knees, the patella experiences contused lacerations, in which the bursa in front of the patella can be injured. This injury can often become chronic and should be treated by a physician. Bone fractures of the lower or upper leg can also occur in falls, although they are much less frequent since the introduction of the clipless pedal.

Anatomy

The knee joint is the largest in the human body and is formed by the junction of three bones: the femur, the tibia, and the patella. It is not a simple hinge joint that works like a door, but also a pivot joint, meaning that as well as flexion and extension, it also enables the lower leg to twist. The ends of the femur, the tibial plateau and the back of the patella, form the surfaces of the knee joint, which are covered with a thick layer of cartilage. As the cartilage surfaces do not fit on top of each other, Mother Nature has invented something very special to ensure that they fit together: the menisci. The meniscus is a wedge-like, half-moon-shaped piece of cartilage that enables the two curved joint surfaces of the femur and tibia to fit together, and it acts as a buffer between these bones. In addition, the meniscus distributes the pressure over a larger cartilage surface, decreasing wear and tear and stabilizing the joint (two menisci per knee). The two cruciate ligaments found in the knee (anterior and posterior) and the two lateral collateral ligaments together create a stable structure. The muscles of the knee enhance the stability; the stronger the thigh and lower leg muscles, the better the knee and ankle joints are protected from injuries.

The patella as a lever

The knee is actually composed of two joints. Next to the joint between the femur and the tibia is the second knee joint, and this occasionally causes problems for cyclists. The patella is embedded in the tendon of the quadriceps and articulates with the patellar surface of the femur; both joints are normally covered with sufficient cartilage. The patella acts as a pulley for the tendons of the quadriceps and increases their strength like a lever.

If the extension muscles are contracted and the leg is straightened, like when pushing on the pedals, the patella slides on the femoral groove.

If, over a protracted period, the pressure on the cartilage is too high or unevenly distributed, the structure of the cartilage changes and a kind of painful inflammation sets in; the cartilage itself is insensitive to pain.

Encapsulated joint

The flexor muscles are attached to the tibia and fibula at the back of the knee. They, too, cause cyclists pain where they are connected to the bones as tendons. Bursae lies under the tendons, muscles, and sometimes skin and protect the sensitive structure of those tissues. The knee contains a number of bursae, which are sensitive to cold because it makes them slightly inflamed. The knee joint is surrounded by a double-layered capsule: an external, taught capsule, which also has a supporting function and an inner capsule that supplies the joint with synovial fluid. Synovial fluid contains nutrients for the joint cartilage and reaches the cartilage through diffusion.

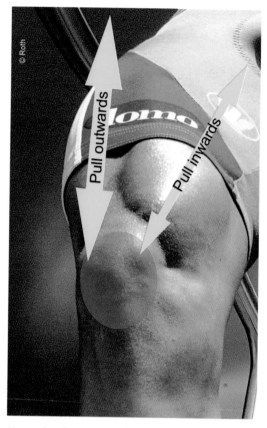

Unequal pull can cause pain.

Longevity

The longevity of the human knee is unsurpassed by that of artificially created joints. In addition, a biological joint can also repair itself if the damage and injury are not too great, which artificial joints cannot yet do.

When your knee hurts!

It is impossible to list the symptoms of knee pain without using medical technical terminology, but these are translated and explained. What in the simplified description at first appears so clear is actually much more complicated; an exact diagnosis and the right treatment is often very difficult to establish due to the many possible factors involved.

1. Kneecap pain

One of the most common knee problems among cyclists is chondromalacia patellae, a degeneration of the cartilage of the underside of the patella. Chondro means cartilage and malacia means softening and patella means kneecap. This softening of the cartilage is accompanied by a change in the microstructure and a nutrient deficiency of the cartilage. In this state of "hunger," the cartilage is unprotected from mechanical wear and tear, resulting in stress pain underneath the patella and in severe cases pain after exercise or even pain at rest.

Many reasons

Chondromalacia patellae is due to a combination of many causes, although most of them can be rectified. Excessive strain, a badly set-up bicycle and cold weather favor the onset of chondromalacia.

Once it has set in, the first thing to do is eliminate these three factors in order to give medical treatment a chance of working.

Raise the saddle. Even a slightly higher saddle can provide relief, as the pressure of the patella on the femur is then reduced and the cartilage can heal. Another cause can be a muscular imbalance between two heads of the quadriceps (musculus vastus lateralis and musculus vastus medialis). As the vastus medialis muscle is not used as much as the vastus lateralis muscle in cycling, the external muscle part of the patella is pulled outward, leading to excessive strain on the outside edge of the patella and possibly to inflammation and wear and tear. For this reason, it is important in physiotherapeutic treatment to strengthen the vastus medialis so that both muscles are equally strong.

2. Tendon inflammations

Tendinopathies are at least as common as chondromalacia. Tendo means tendon and pathy means disease, specifically an inflammation of the tendon, its insertion into the bone, and its transition to the muscle. The following are susceptible to tendinopathies:

a. The patellar tendon, where it is joined by the tibia and where the patella originates
b. The quadriceps tendon
c. The head of the tibula
d. The tendons of the flexors at the inside of the back of the knee. If the latter are affected, it often helps to lower the height of the saddle, which lessens the strong pull of the muscles and tendons. The upper edge of the patella at the insertion of the quadriceps is often affected by tendinopathy. Symptoms are pain at rest and

during exercise in the affected place. Causes can again be cold weather and excessive strain and also incorrectly adjusted pedals and the occasional incompatibility of fixed pedal systems. Stretching is advisable in order to keep the muscles and tendons flexible and supple. In particular, this often stops the onset of irritation of the tendons and muscles in the knee area.

Other causes

In all symptoms, however, there are also causes that are not related to cycling. A difference in leg length (should be compensated for in the cycling shoes) or pelvic obliquity, bow-legs or bandy-legs, flat feet, and prior damage to the knees or ankles can provoke the same sports injuries and damage as in the points listed. If pain does occur (the body's early warning sign), you should start by checking the relevant points, and if self-treatment doesn't work, seek out a sports physician with cycling experience.

3. Bursitis

Another knee problem caused mainly by cold weather is bursitis, or the inflammation of the bursa, which can be extremely painful if left untreated. The bursa in front of the patella, normally not noticeable, is most commonly affected; it swells up and hurts with every step.

Providing relief

The main causes for musculoskeletal pain, in particular the knee, are explained next. Before consulting a physician, these points should be checked.

1. Pedal in low gears

Although the impact on the knees is low, famous cycling stars like Bernard Hinault or Stephen Roche were forced to end their careers because they were plagued by severe knee pain. In the case of these professionals, the reason for their knee problems was almost certainly excessively high gear ratios such as 53 x 12 or more and excessive strain for years on end. Consequently, low to medium gears should be used as often as possible, particularly in the preparation phase. Misusing high gears can lead to pain in the tendon and muscle insertions, and if these gears are used for many years, the result can be the development of irreparable joint damage. Plenty of amateurs and professionals can tolerate this type of strain, but they must not. However, if you are the type who reacts sensitively to biomechanical stress, then take care.

2. Keeping warm

The second error that recreational cyclists, and even occasionally experienced cyclists, make is not protecting their muscles and joints well enough from the cold. For example, they cycle in shorts when the weather is too cold. Apart from the fact that the muscles cool down and you can easily pull a muscle or catch a cold, it is very damaging to the knees. As the knee contains very little subcutaneous tissue, and as the bones, tendons, and ligaments lie directly below the skin, the knee gets cold very quickly. These structures often become inflamed in the following days. If the bursa is affected, the pain can become chronic. The cartilage also gets cold so that it is even more poorly supplied with nutrients than before, and the entire knee metabolism slows down and the cartilage loses elasticity. If this kind of exposure to the cold is repeated often, and on top of this, high gear ratios are used, microscopic changes can take place in the cartilage resulting in a loss of smoothness in the top surface. A joint with cartilage defects no longer functions smoothly, and wear and tear damage is inevitable.

Shorts From 68 °F

You should always keep your legs warm when cycling and do not remove long trousers or tights until the temperature hits 65-68 °F. Unwisely, most cyclists always race in shorts irrespective of the weather conditions. However, this is now changing. In recent years, knee warmers and cropped cycling tights are used more and more often to keep the knees warm. If you still want to race with bare knees, cover them with a thick layer of oil or fat to protect them just before they start to cool down (see Massage). Although often recommended, heating pads do not even come near to being as effective as knee warmers and can even be damaging, as all they do is increase the blood supply. On day rides, it is advisable to wear knee warmers or knee tights that can be easily removed while riding on cold mornings.

3. Sitting position

Your sitting position on the bike is another factor that must be checked. If it is too high or too low, it negatively affects your pedaling action. The knees must bend a lot more if the saddle height is too low and the pressure on the joint structures, particularly the patella, are consequently higher than with a correctly set-up saddle. Likewise a saddle that is too high—meaning the legs are fully extended when pedaling—can cause problems mainly for the hamstrings and back. However, a slightly higher sitting position is recommended for cyclists with patella problems, as this reduces pressure peaks on the sensitive areas.

4. Pedal system

Finally, the pedal system should be checked, because a bent shoe plate can be very damaging for joints and muscles. If you stop and think how many times your legs must bend and straighten during a just even a 60 km bike tour—about 10,000 times—you will realize the importance of correctly adjusted shoe plates. The feet normally pedal parallel to the pedal cranks, and you should never get an uncomfortable feeling in your joints. If you don't get on with fixed clipless pedal systems that do not allow the foot to move from side to side, you should consider a flexible system such as those manufactured by TIME. These do not restrict the natural rotation of the ankle and foot; without the exertion of force, the foot can only turn the pedal a few degrees before the pedal is released.

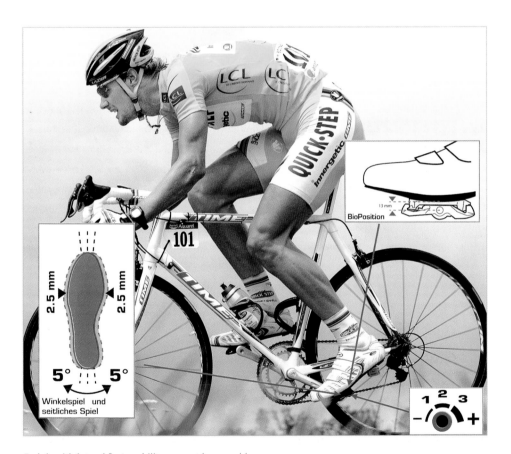

Pedals with lateral foot mobility prevent knee problems

Insoles

It is possible to counteract the rotation caused by fallen arches in order to reduce the pain; this involves an inward rotation of the ankle (when the leg straightens) caused by the foot arch falling when it is placed under greater strain. Supporting the arch with a custom-made orthopedic insole stops the arch from falling when the leg is straightened and the rotation that causes the pain is reduced. One manufacturer of cycling shoes now sells shoes with pre-prepared insoles for different foot types or offers the possibility of adapting the shoe to the foot with a removable wedge.

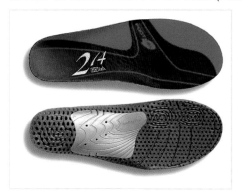

Customized insoles prevent fallen arches.

5. Bent bicycle parts

Bike accidents often lead to bent cranks and pedal axles, which make the feet deviate from the ideal circular path and place them under strains that they may be able to tolerate in the short-term but not in the long-term. The misalignment extends from the ankle to the knee and hip and can ultimately even be the cause of back pain.

c) Foot

The main problems affecting the foot area are inflammations of the Achilles tendon. The Achilles tendon connects the calf muscle to the heel bone, and its exposed position on the heel means that the tendon is vulnerable to the cold. Incorrect sitting positions, cold (lack of overshoes), or overuse (gears too high) often cause irritation that can turn into inflammation. All these factors must be considered in the case of Achilles tendonitis.

In the case of an insertional Achilles **tendonitis**, the **tendon junctions** with the muscle or bone are inflamed.

Treatment: Change the above-mentioned factors and have physiotherapy.

Cyclists may find the tendons of the front shin muscle (tibialis anterior) hurt particularly after racing in cold, wet conditions. Treatment is the same as already mentioned.

Hot Foot (Metatarsalgia)

Burning or painful soles can have several causes. Laces or Velcro that are fastened too tightly can restrict blood circulation in the feet, causing pain. Also, a very hard insole can promote the burning sensation; a thin but soft and well-fitting insole will provide relief. In addition, the soles of the cycling shoes should be anatomically shaped as a flat sole encourages the arch to drop, which can cause pain in the sole of the foot (plantar fasciitis) and the knee.

d) Back

The back muscles enable the cyclist to pedal hard even though they are not directly involved in the pedaling action. They stabilize the body and improve the transfer of power from the legs to the pedals. The term backache covers a whole multitude of complaints and symptoms in which muscles, ligaments, joints, and joint capsules and tendons can all be affected and cause pain. Studies show that about 30-50% of all racing cyclists complain of back pain or admit to having suffered from them at some point in their career. This percentage corresponds to that of the non-cycling population.

There is a difference between **local pain**, which does not radiate into other areas, and **pseudo-radicular pain**. The latter can radiate into the leg or the head and even cause sensation disorder in severe cases. Slipped discs occur only rarely while cycling, but their onset can be hastened by cycling.

High Gears

Cycling in high gears (e.g., 52 x 12) puts a lot of pressure on the lumbar vertebrae and on the joints and other structures of the lumbar spine. So much so that degenerative changes (wear and tear) can result if the preconditions for it exist.

Beginners, in particular, may also have other causes for back pain. An incorrectly set-up bike for example can cause aches and pains very quickly, and if it is adjusted and set up correctly, these aches and pains usually disappear equally quickly. Both racing cyclists and beginners may complain of back pain particularly at the start of the racing season. This is due to a lack of suppleness and poor muscle fitness. In winter, but also in summer, a reduction in skin temperature can be another cause of pain, although this can be reduced by wearing appropriate clothing.

Weak Abs

An imbalance between the muscles of the abdomen and back alters the statics of the spinal column and therefore may be the cause of pain. As a rule, cyclists have poorly developed abdominal muscles. A strength imbalance between the left and right legs can also cause back pain. Back pain can become a vicious cycle in which tension in the muscles can lead to other tensions. In order to break this cycle, the primary causes must be identified and corrected instead of just treating the symptoms. There are also many other causes of back pain to be considered that are not caused by cycling.

Treatment

In each of the previously mentioned cases, spinal exercises, general core strengthening exercises (see chapters 3.8 and 3.9), physical therapy, and massage are effective treatments. A stretching program, as presented in chapter 3.9, often solves the problem in a matter of days. However, it is also important to wear functional underwear, to ride in low gears, and to check your sitting position, as large differences between saddle and handlebar height encourage back pain. Athletes with serious problems in the lumbar spine area are therefore advised to bring their saddle and handlebar to a height at which pressure is taken away from the structures and can, for example, be done very successfully by means of a slightly upward-pointing stem or spacers in the headset. Furthermore, tires with greater cushioning (25 mm, max. 6 bar) should be used instead of hard racing tires. Athletes who have already suffered from a serious back injury (e.g., slipped disc) must proceed with extreme caution and pursue the rest of their sporting career under the supervision of a physician experienced in treating cyclists.

e) Neck

Neck pain is not that common among cyclists. Due to the position on the bike, the natural hyperextension (lordosis) of the cervical spine is exaggerated, particularly when your hands are "on the drops." If the stem is also too long or the handlebar–saddle height difference is too great, the neck must be hyperextended even further in order to be able to see the road.

This often causes pain in the back of the neck and the upper back, which are usually muscle origins. Particularly at the beginning of the racing season and in beginners, the muscles of the back of the neck (trapezius, small neck muscles) cramp up due to their lack of fitness and produce pain, which does disappear though after a few weeks of training. These muscles, which support the head weighing an average of 15 lb, mainly work statically (isometrically). In other words, they don't move but just exercise a supporting function. The isometric contraction closes the blood vessels in the muscles, thus reducing their blood supply. This results in a painful, cramp-like situation.

Pain Relief

Relief can only be obtained by moving the areas concerned, by regular stretching and frequent changes of position on the bike, in order to improve the blood supply to the tissues. This also applies to the back. As well as the specific mobilizing of the back and neck, there are other measures that can alleviate or prevent neck pain. A lighter helmet (0.5 lb) puts a lot less strain on the neck muscles than an older, heavier helmet. High neck vests and jerseys protect the neck from cold airstreams. When cycling, your arms should always be slightly bent, never straight, so that they can absorb bumps in the road like shock absorbers.

f) Head

As the scalp can get cold very quickly, for example in descents or in the winter, headaches are common. They can be avoided by wearing a beanie hat under the helmet, which also protects you from catching a cold or sunstroke. If you do not wear good quality UV protecting sunglasses during bright, sunny weather (especially in the mountains or on the coast), cramped eye muscles caused by squinting may lead to head and neck aches.

The head and neck are particularly vulnerable in falls and collisions. Varying degrees of concussion are often the result of falling onto your head. In the worst case, a fall can lead to a fractured skull, which is the most serious injury a cyclist can experience.

Fortunately, fractured skulls or necks are extremely rare. More common are dislocated cervical vertebrae, broken noses, broken or dislocated jaws, or skin abrasions. Less common is the degenerative wear and tear of the small vertebral joints of the cervical spine.

g) Shoulder and arm

In the shoulder area, fractures are the most frequent injury. The collar bone connects the shoulder joint (upper arm, shoulder blade, collar bone) to the breastbone and also, via the ribs, to the spine. It is therefore the only fixed link from the arm to the torso. When you land on your shoulder, hand, or elbow in a fall, the collarbone is placed under such great pressure that it often cannot withstand, and it breaks. Even the strong collarbone ligaments can tear. As the recovery process lasts about five months, professional cyclists often have operations to accelerate healing so that they can get back in the saddle as soon as possible. Apart from possible falls and their consequences, the shoulder area causes very few problems in cycling. Fall injuries in the shoulder area can be effectively reduced by a strong muscle corset around the shoulder joint. Push-ups are an ideal exercise for this.

Tensions, which are often caused by cramped neck muscles, can often appear in the shoulder during long training rides. This can be dealt with by targeted exercises, riding with the elbows slightly bent and checking the sitting position.

h) Hands

Because holding the handlebars while cycling places the forearm muscles under great strain, partly caused by a tight grip, both elbows are prone to tennis elbow caused by the pull of the tendons in the forearm muscles.

This can usually be alleviated by a cycling ban, rest, and physiotherapy. The grip on the handlebar should be relaxed as often as possible, and varied and the different grips should be used. Now and then, take the hands off the handlebar altogether and move them around. This also helps to avoid the common problem of cyclist or handlebar palsy when nerve lesions in the hand area cause symptoms ranging from numb fingers to paralysis. This involves a squeezing of the nerves and blood vessels in the carpal tunnel in the wrist and can be alleviated by padded gloves and handlebars with a wide grip or double-wrapped handlebars.

The wrist and indeed the whole arm are very vulnerable in falls, as a falling cyclist's reflex is almost always to try to break the fall with his hands. Despite gloves, the palms of the hands are often injured. More serious than this kind of skin injury are the wrist, forearm, and upper arm fractures that can be sustained during falls onto the arms.

© Roth

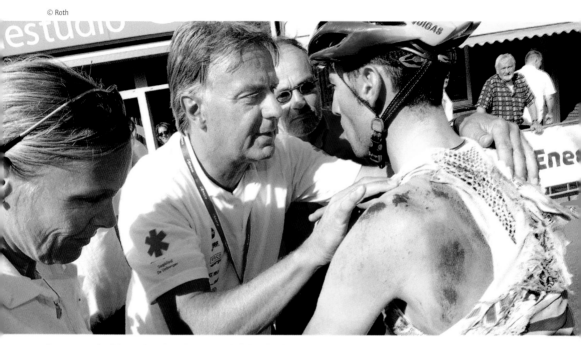

Grazes may look harmless, but they are painful and take time to heal.

6.3   Skin Damage and Injuries

Grazes caused by falls

Grazes are the main skin injuries caused by falls. Grazes are unfortunately part of the cyclist's daily life, and they usually occur on the hip (thigh), knee (lower leg), shoulder, and elbow. The wounds are often located in places on which we sleep and which are constantly being bent and stretched. If large areas are affected, it is advisable to make a frame (e.g., a kind of leg cage) that stops the sheets from touching the skin in the affected spot when you are sleeping. Cyclists must absolutely ensure that their tetanus injections are up to date, as even falls that cause light grazes can often bring you into contact with sources of tetanus. Contrary to rumor, tetanus injections do not harm performance.

Shaved legs

Shaved legs are also a necessity for racing cyclists, as wounds on hairy skin heal more slowly and hurt more, because the hairs irritate the wounds. It also allows wounds to be treated more easily, because in falls, dirt always enters the wound and must be removed when the wound is treated afterward. If the wound is not too deep, it can be cleaned with disinfectant, but deeper wounds should be treated by a physician.

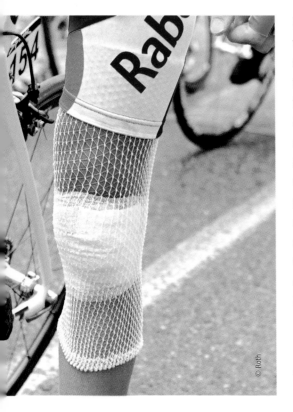

© Roth

It is always advisable to wipe the cleaned wound with a suitable disinfectant to protect it from possible infection. Smaller wounds can then be left without a dressing, while larger ones need further treatment. First cover the clean surface with Desitin® and then with a gel compress (non-stick) or a Vaseline cloth. Then place some sterile gauze or the combined dressing can also be covered with plaster to stop it from slipping. The dressing should be changed daily. In this way, the wound remains soft and flexible, and the sensitive scab cannot even form at first and usually after just a few weeks the new skin has grown. Modern wound dressings perform the same function as the described ointment dressings.

If a solid scab has already formed over the wound, it is best to leave it without a dressing. Deeper cuts definitely need to be treated, and possibly stitched, by a physician.

Seat area

The seat can sometimes be painful due to friction soreness as well as the pressure that the skin and the structures underneath it are subject to. Other causes of saddle soreness may be a badly padded hard saddle, uneven road surface, and lack of hygiene. Boils and even carbuncles (multiple boils) are formed because sweat and bacteria on the surface of the skin are rubbed into the skin made sensitive by friction and infect the roots of the fine hairs (hair follicle infection).

This shows the importance of hygiene in this area, which also involves wearing clean cycling tights that are changed almost daily. Rubbing the bottom with a special cream, Vaseline, or Desitin before a ride likewise helps to maintain an infection-free seat. Once an infection has set in, a hip bath followed by rubbing in a commercially available seat cream, better still with Desitin. Boils are treated with blistering ointment. Careful prevention with the appropriate treatment is very important in order to avoid the development of abscesses and other infections.

Sunburn

A cyclist's skin is exposed to strong sunshine, especially in the summer months. It is often forgotten that several hours spent on the bike in short tights and a short-sleeved jersey can cause sunburn just as much as lying on the beach. The UV radiation in the mountains is already significantly higher than on the flat, which can lead to serious burns. As well as sunburn, UV radiation can also have other negative consequences for the skin:

1. skin ageing,

2. carcinoma (skin cancer), and

3. allergic and toxic reactions (sun allergies).

For these reasons, you should apply an appropriate suntan lotion before training rides in the summer, especially as UV radiation has increased considerably in recent years due to the hole in the ozone layer. Existing sunburned skin should be carefully protected by clothing (gloves, oversleeves, leggings). It has been shown that cyclists' skin reacts particularly sensitively to the sun at spring training camps (February/March) and not infrequently even has an allergic reaction to the unfamiliar strength of the sun. These cyclists can take preventive calcium preparations in order to avoid possible allergies at training camp (in consultation with a physician).

White and pasty

Cyclists must bear in mind when they expose their skin to the sun in the summer that their arms and legs are already used to the sun and tanned, while the skin of the upper body that is normally covered with clothes can burn very easily. A severe burn can make you feel very ill, possibly even feverish, and also cause your performance to deteriorate.

6.4   Various Medical Topics

Numbness

In men, high pressure combined with high numbers of shocks and bumps (poor road surfaces) can cause swelling of the prostate, a compression lesion of the urethra, or nerve and vascular compression can lead to numbness in the penis, pain when urinating (urethra), and possibly even blood in the urine or in a very rare case to cause temporary impotence.

A break from training for a few days will get rid of even the most stubborn symptoms of these typical cycling complaints. Relief can be obtained by a special anatomically-shaped softer and possibly slightly forward-leaning saddle, wider well-cushioned tires, and a slightly higher handle-bar. You should also stand up out of the saddle regularly while cycling in order to take the pressure off the seat and the sensitive areas underneath it (prostate, ureter, nerves, spermatic duct).

Impotence

In the worst case, cycling can cause temporary impotence due to a pressure lesion on the nerves, although regular, moderate cycling is beneficial for sex life. It has been established, though, that heavy endurance exercise leads to a drop in testosterone levels (male sex hormone), which can be a cause of sexual problems.

Performance levels and menstruation

A change in performance levels has been observed during the female menstrual cycle, al-though not all women are affected equally. In cycling, it is typical for performance levels to de-teriorate during menstruation. Taking the contraceptive pill can stabilize performance in many cases, although the pill does have other side-effects (e.g., weight gain, loss of speed, psycholo-gical complications). Regular endurance exercise over many years may result in cycles without ovulation combined with amenorrhoea (lack of menstrual periods). Some top female cyclists go for years without menstruating. Sports-related changes in the hormone balance are responsible for this, and they are reversible. In a normal cycle, the monthly blood loss and heavy exercise often cause anemia, which can be managed with an appropriate diet and, if necessary, the addition of iron supplements.

Performance-limiting medication

There is a whole range of medication that can negatively impact cycling performance. When taking medication, always discuss with your physician whether it is wise to exercise in view of the type of illness and medication concerned. In many cases, cycling should be avoided until health is restored. These are some medicines that harm performance levels: sleeping tablets, high blood pressure medication, cold remedies, allergy medication, and muscle-relaxants. In the case of long-term medication, get advice as to whether it is safe to practice sports at the same time. It is also important to ensure that any medication you take does not infringe doping guidelines.

Head colds and cycling

Training rides in cold and windy weather make cyclists very vulnerable to catching colds. Cyclists should take great care to protect themselves from head colds and infections, particularly in the preparation phase and at the start of the racing phase in April, when the weather may be poor. Very heavy training and racing can compromise the immune system thereby increasing susceptibility to infection. Training with a heavy head cold or even fever is out of the question, as other organs may be affected (e.g., the heart). Following recovery, training should be resumed gradually. If the return to training is too fast, it can lead to a state of overtraining.

Give yourself time to recover!

After a heavy, one-week head cold, it will take at least two to three weeks to regain the same performance level as before. If sniffles are ignored, this can lead to chronic sinus problems or even suppurative frontal sinusitis, which must definitely be cured before training can be resumed, as this kind of suppurative focus can harbor a risk of heart damage. To protect yourself from respiratory infections, it is sensible to wear weather-appropriate cycling clothing, which should be removed as fast as possible after training. A warm winter beanie hat stops the head from cooling down after racing and training. A diet rich in vitamins and minerals helps to stabilize the immune system, as do regular saunas. In training camps, during which the immune system is usually quite vulnerable, do not share drinking bottles in order to avoid spreading germs. It can happen that an infection (gastric flu or head cold) can put a whole training group out of action.

Allergies (hay fever)

Spring is torture for cyclists who suffer from hay fever. At this time of year, the air is full of different types of pollen so that for allergic cyclists training is impossible, never mind racing. If the allergy is severe, desensitization treatments are recommended, in which the aim is to develop the patient's immunity by means of increasing doses of pollen injections. After the first year of treatment, a tangible improvement is usually felt. As well as desensitization, antihistamine medication can also be taken to combat allergies, although they are really strong and have such a strong effect on the body that performance levels drop significantly. For a few cyclists, the allergies (which can appear from one year to the next) mean the end of their career.

6.5 Overtraining

Overtraining means an overloading of the body characterized by symptoms of chronic fatigue. Unlike acute fatigue after training, this is a permanent condition that features a number of symptoms.

Little is known about how it originates, particularly in cycling. One thing that is certain is that recovery is impaired in an athlete suffering from overtraining. There are two different types of overtraining: **parasympathetic overtraining**, which often affects endurance athletes, and **sympathetic overtraining**. These names correspond to the two components of the vegetative nervous system (see chapter 2.1).

Parasympathetic overtraining involves an inhibited state of arousal, whereas sympathetic over-training involves overexcitation.

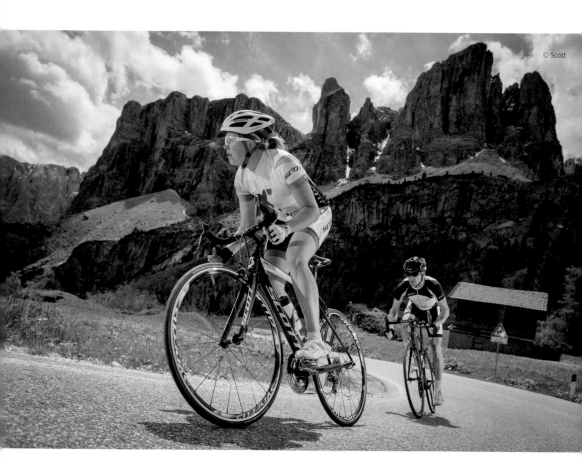

© Scott

Chronic Fatigue

Parasympathetic overtraining is common in cycling and is hard to diagnose, as it develops gradually and its symptoms are the same as those of normal exhaustion. A great deal of experience is required to realize the difference between the two and make an accurate diagnosis. A blood test can confirm a suspected case of overtraining by identifying raised levels of urea and creatine kinase concentrations at rest. The exercise lactate concentration and heart rate values are low, which may be incorrectly interpreted as a result of improved performance capacity. Table 6.1 lists the symptoms of both overtraining states.

Overtraining is usually a result of a training or racing load that is too high or a completely wrong training program. In parasympathetic overtraining, training intensity has a greater influence on the state of overtraining than training volume.

The first thing to do is reduce the training intensity. Psychological stress can also promote the onset of overtraining, especially if the psychological stress is related to cycling, and you find it almost impossible to switch off.

Table 6.1: Overtraining

Parasympathetic overtraining	Sympathetic overtraining
• Fatigue	• Fatigue
• Reduced performance	• Reduced performance
• Inhibition	• Excitement
• Lower resting heart rate	• Higher resting heart rate
• Lower maximal heart rate	• Slower dropping of heart rate after exercise
• Normal or increased need for sleep	• Insomnia and sleeplessness
• Bad mood and depression	• Restlessness and irritability
• Normal appetite	• Loss of appetite
• Constant bodyweight	• Weight loss
• Increased training due to reduced performance	• Reluctance to train
• Increased risk of infection	• Increased risk of infection
• Lack of glycogen	• Palpitations

Treating overtraining

The treatment of overtraining depends on its characteristics, as a few days' rest often sufficiently allow the body to recover in mild forms with light symptoms. Severe forms need weeks
or even months of adapted training preceded by a break from training of at least a week.
Then, training should be resumed at greatly reduced intensity and lower volumes, with no
racing at all, and training should only be increased after consistent improvement. A mental
break from cycling is also necessary.

Recovery measures such as sauna, massage, stretching, and also mental recovery and relaxation are crucial in the treatment of overtraining. As this state is often accompanied by reduced
muscle glycogen levels, a balanced, high-carbohydrate diet is also essential. In any case, it is
advisable to consult a physician with experience in endurance sports.

6.6   Doping

Doping is improving performance using banned methods. The desire to improve human performance by secretive means is as old as mankind itself. Even athletes in Ancient Greece and
Rome used "magic potions" and precious substances that were intended to give them greater
strength. As another example, the Incas in South America ran about 400 miles in three days
under the influence of cocaine, an unbelievable performance that was not only due to the consumption of cocaine but also has its roots in a religious sacrifice. Then, as now, the belief in a
certain method was very important, for many substances have no effect at all and even harm
the athlete. If any effect is noticed, it is usually a placebo effect.

A long tradition of doping

Cycling has been a classic doping event since its early days, so it is not surprising that for a
very long time, doping has been a completely normal process for many racing cyclists. Luckily,
society now views doping as immoral, and the practice is outlawed as much as possible. However, this applies only partially to cycling, even though it is the sport with the most caught
doping offenders, and even this only represents the tip of the iceberg, as the true figure is
undoubtedly much higher. The long-distance race from Bordeaux to Paris in 1886 saw the first
death from doping.

The most prominent doping victim was definitely the English cyclist Tom Simpson, who
collapsed just before the peak when climbing Mont Ventoux during the Tour de France on

July 13, 1967 and died shortly afterward. It is precisely those sports that were professional in the beginning (e.g., cycling, boxing), and in which relatively large sums of money could be won, that had the biggest doping problem, and unfortunately this is still the case.

How does doping happen?

Doping methods are mainly popularized by word-of-mouth recommendation, as there are very few studies on the sporting effects of the substances on the anti-doping list. Often, cyclists are encouraged by their coaches to take a certain "performance-enhancing" substance. However, the problem with this is that almost nobody, neither cyclist nor coach, possesses the necessary knowledge to be able to assess the effect of the drugs, much less any possible side effects or long-term consequences. In many cases, the drug does not even achieve the aim of performance enhancement. This short-sighted behavior, which is only focused on achieving short-term success with absolutely no regard for the athlete's future (long-term consequences), is unfortunately very hard to stop.

Drugs tests

In cycling, drug tests only take place at big races and circuits; in the smaller circuit races that often offer good prize money, doping disappears into a gray area and can be undertaken with only minimal risk of discovered. The problem with drug testing is that tests are very expensive, and at the moment it is impossible to test every athlete so that only the very top cyclists are tested. The effectiveness of many drug tests must be questioned, according to some professional cyclists who have confessed to doping. Performance-enhancing substances are even often used in recreational and grass-roots cycling (cyclosportives).

Substance classes

The main substances used in cycling are those that prolong or enhance endurance and reduce the associated pain. Drugs that stimulate the athlete are called **stimulants**. They may often even be addictive. As well as amphetamines, caffeine is also used as a stimulant, which is completely harmless in small doses, but high doses do have side effects.

Pain is suppressed with **narcotics**, which are available in very different forms and are commonly used as they are so easy to get a hold of. Apart from the not insignificant side effects of narcotics and stimulants, the danger of taking these substances is that they enable performance reserves that are normally protected to be tapped, thus overloading the body and placing the cyclist in great danger and greatly reducing receptivity, coordination, and responsiveness.

The third group of substances used in cycling are **anabolic steroids**, which are related to the male sex hormone testosterone. Anabolic steroids improve strength and the ability to recover as they build more muscle mass. The list of side effects range from an increased risk of injury to kidney and liver damage and an increase in blood lipid levels to infertility.

A banned method of increasing performance is **blood doping**. Widespread in the 1970s, it is now undergoing a renaissance, because it is very effective and is more difficult to detect than doping with EPO (Erythropoietin).

There are illnesses that require medication (e.g., cough syrup) that contain substances that are on the doping list. When you are prescribed these medicines, you should avoid racing out of fairness and to protect your own health. However, affected cyclists are able to start after obtaining permission. Illness is frequently used as an excuse for taking banned substances.

What can be done about doping in cycling?

A key factor in reducing doping is information, particularly in a traditionally doping-tainted sport like cycling. Only when both athletes and coaches are informed of the medical dangers and the moral reprehensibility of doping can the problem be solved. The key to a doping-free sport lies in prevention work with young people, replacing officials, and stricter punishment of doping offenders.

Drugs tests, particularly in smaller races, can set the necessary example and support this. If you know cyclists who occasionally resort to doping, you should react to this and if necessary report them to the anti-doping authorities who can then carry out *targeted drug tests*. However, there will probably always be athletes in all sports who try to gain an advantage over their opponents by using banned methods.

6.7   Massage

Massage is a technique for relieving tension and pain that dates back to ancient times and is in fact the oldest form of medical treatment. Particularly at professional and top amateur level, the soigneur—the cycling assistant—is irreplaceable, as he not only gives massage treatments but also looks after the cyclists in other ways.

He is also a kind of psychologist who listens to the cyclist and helps him to think about things differently. This makes it obvious that, as well as being important from a physiological and mechanical point of view, the mental relaxation aspect is also very valuable for athletes.

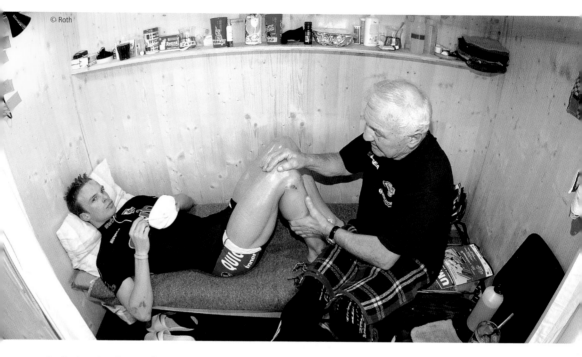

Professional cyclists receive regular massages, often daily during tours.

A good masseur can tell by feeling a cyclist's legs how good he is, as the skin thickness, the amount of connective tissue, and the suppleness of the muscles are indicative of the performance level and type of cyclist.

There are three different forms of cycling massage that are differentiated according to when they are used and the type of massage:

1. Training massage: used after an intensive workout, usually during the week

2. Race massage: used before a race to relax and improve the blood circulation to the muscles as part of the warm-up program

3. Recovery massage: used after a race to speed up recovery and relaxation

Massage effects

- The mechanical treatment of the body brings about an increase in **blood circulation** both in the skin and in the muscles, although this absolutely does not mean that a massage can replace the warm-up, as is still sometimes falsely stated.

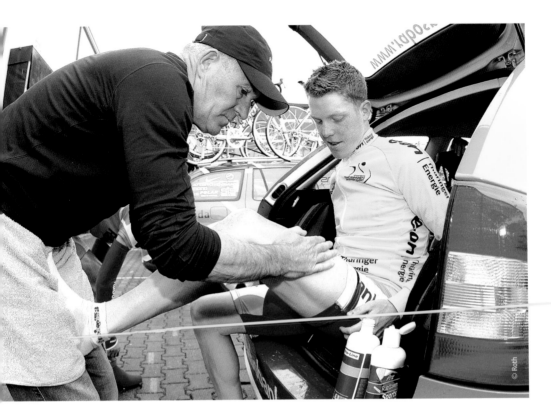

- **Tension** and **knots** can be gotten rid of with the aid of massage. Massage calms the nervous system via the nerve endings and also helps promote organ function.
- It reduces the **heart and breathing rates**.
- New research calls into question and even partly denies the **increased elimination of metabolic waste**.
- One of the most important effects of massage is the psychological effect, as it feels good, promotes well-being, increases mental preparedness (for the race to follow), and also promotes relaxation and recovery.

What to look for in a cycling massage

First, the massage should take place in a room that is a comfortable temperature with no drafts and not too brightly lit to ensure optimal relaxation for the cyclist. This is not the place to explore exact massage techniques, as this should be reserved for experts with many years of experience. However, here are a few tips that can help a masseur who has little experience with cycling to give a good cycling massage. It is important not just to concentrate on the most important part of the cyclist's body, the legs, but also to include the back, the back of the neck, and the shoulders in order to loosen any tension in these areas. The leg massage should be done very gently, as the muscles here are usually extremely sensitive and should therefore consist mainly of strokes, gentle kneading, and shaking. The normal massage technique would be much too rough for the cyclist's thin skin. Avoid pain during the massage, apart from a few exceptions (muscle knots). A massage done with a lot of pressure and sharp fingers will at best result in sore leg muscles.

Shaved legs, essential for racing cyclists, make the masseur's job a lot easier and also provide protection from painful infected hair follicles and pulled hairs. Different oil mixtures can be used for massage, but a simple baby oil is sufficient. After the massage, remove as much oil as possible with alcohol or liniment to avoid blocking the pores.

The masseur should wait for the athlete to start talking and not insist if he would prefer to remain silent. If you do talk, it is the task of the masseur to direct the conversation away from cycling, particularly after a race, to make the cyclist think of other things.

Self-massage

Self-massage is an excellent, cheap way of relaxing the muscles, especially if you cannot afford expensive visits to the masseur. However, the massage is less relaxing, and you also need to do it yourself. Due to the restricted reach of the arms, self-massage is restricted to the legs and possibly the arms. Self-massage can be done both before and after training and racing. If a recovery massage is performed after exercise, it is advisable to do a stretching program, as described in chapter 3.9, in order pre-relax the mind and muscles. You should learn the following massage technique and use it after heavy exercise, and a shortened form can also be used to relax the muscles. About 10 to 15 minutes is required for massaging both legs.

Where should you do it?

The best place for a self-massage is the soles of the feet. You spread out a towel and sit on it. Before a race, sit in the car or on a curbstone.

What do you need?

For a massage you need one or more towels, massage oil, and some alcohol or liniment in order to remove the oil at the end. Baby oil has been shown to work well. Special massage oils can obviously also be used. If you are preparing your legs for a race, the choice of oil will depend on the weather. If it's cold, a layer of warming oil or cream is recommended. If it is also raining, the legs can then be rubbed with a special warming cream with another layer of oil on top. However, the heating effect of the cream should not be so great that it draws too much blood from the muscles in order to supply blood to the skin. Thermal oils and creams should be avoided as their effect is too superficial. On warm and hot days, no cream should be rubbed in, as this would even prevent heat dissipation.

How do you do it?

As mentioned, the massage should be preceded by a little stretching. Then put your feet up on a wall for a few minutes to improve the venous return. If you prefer the massage to come first, sit on the towel with bare legs and feet and relax as much as possible. The different massage techniques are described in order next.

1. Feet and ankles

You should always start a massage in the parts of the body farthest from the heart and work toward the heart. While you are massaging the first leg, cover the other one with a spare towel to stop it from getting cold. Spread a little oil onto the thigh and lower leg, and use the rest of the oil sticking to the hand for the foot. Start by placing the ankle on the other thigh and rubbing it hard with both hands in order to warm it up. Then pull the knuckles firmly over the sole of the foot in order to stimulate the reflex zones there. A hard object can also be used. Knead each individual toe with the fingers and stretch the arch out both lengthwise and crossways. Then move on to the ankle, working it with circling movements of the fingertips. Afterward, massage up the lower leg beyond the knee with both hands.

2. Achilles tendon

Run the Achilles tendon with light strokes and knead with the foot cocked. Stretching during the massage is particularly beneficial.

3. Calf

Start a calf massage with repeated light strokes of the lower leg toward the heart. Then use many small strokes from bottom to top and then knead a little to slowly loosen the calf muscles. Now and then, smooth the lower leg out and shake the calf between the hands.

4. Shin muscles

Rub the shin muscles, located on the outside of the lower leg, a few times with the backs of the fists. The edge of the shin bone situated on the inside of the lower leg should not be massaged as it is not only painful but can also cause inflammation in the long term.

5. Knee

Rub and stroke around the knee very gently with the fingers, exerting very little pressure.

6. Quadriceps

After stroking and shaking the calf, turn your attention to the thigh. Here, too, the massage starts with hard, two-handed stroking and shaking that are repeated occasionally. With the leg straight, massage each muscle part of the quadriceps from the insertion at the knee to the origin in the hip flexor. The insertions in particular should be carefully loosened with many small, light kneading movements.

7. Hamstrings

The backs of the thigh are hard to reach in a DIY massage, although they can be shaken very easily. With the leg bent and the foot on the floor, lightly knead the muscles and stroke them with the palm of the hand. The insertions of the hamstring in the back of the knee can be accessed easily when the knee is bent.

A few stretching exercises also support the effect of the massage. Before turning your attention to the other leg, cover the previously massaged leg with a towel. Allow five to eight minutes to massage each leg. Hardened spots or knots in the muscles should not be smoothed out with brute strength. Such tense areas require more time, and careful kneading and rubbing often get rid of the hardening.

After the massage, remove the surplus oil from the legs, and then put your feet up. After the regenerative massage, the muscles should not be overly strained by standing up for long periods. Once you have some experience of DIY massage, you can even carefully massage a training partner (e.g., at a training camp); as long as you remember that a massage should not hurt and should be an enjoyable experience, you cannot go wrong.

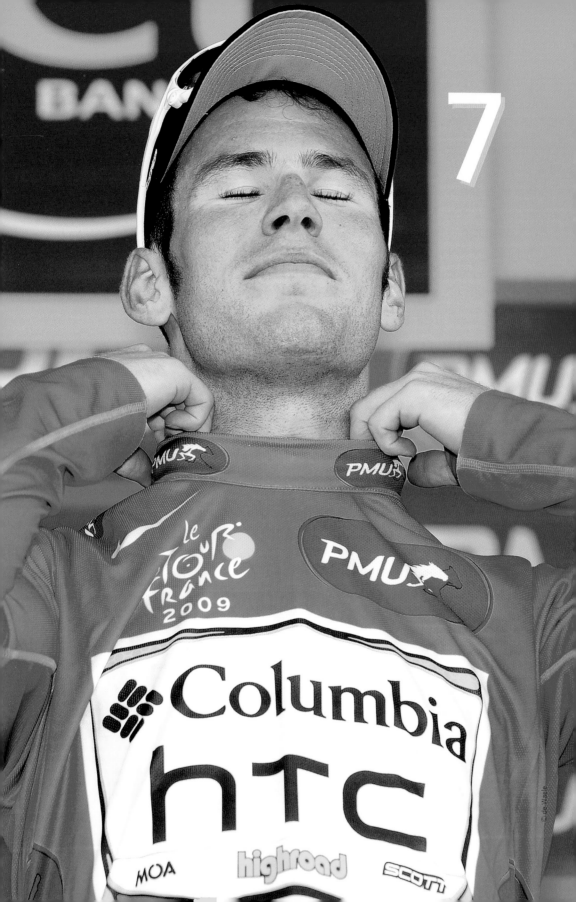

7   Psychology

7.1   Introduction

Behind the rather mysterious sounding term sports psychology hides an interdisciplinary science that is concerned with the identification, explanation, and application of psychological factors that influence sports performance. However, at this point we are less interested in the scientific and theological side of cycling psychology and more interested in maintaining or improving performance with the aid of practical tips. For this reason, this chapter starts with an initial, brief insight into this highly interesting topic and ends with a few recommended exercises (mental race preparation). There is a wealth of further reading available on the topic of sports psychology.

Mental strength

There are those in sporting circles who still assume that a strong body leads to a strong mind, but we now know that in fact the opposite is true. In a long sprint or a mountaintop finish, it is always the indomitable will that drives the cyclist on despite the pain in his legs that would otherwise have caused him to drop out long before. Out of two equally strong cyclists who also use the same equipment, the one with the greater mental strength will always prevail. With very sophisticated and monitored physical training at high performance level, psychological training is one of the few ways of ensuring performance improvement or at least performance stabilization in the future once doping is gone. This is why, in a number of sports, athletes are able to achieve peak performances with the aid of different forms of mental training. In particular, sports in which extreme, short-lived concentration can make the difference between victory and defeat. For example, in high jump, 100 m, and shooting, rapid progress can be made with psychological training. The same is true for martial arts. Anyone who is successful in any sport at the highest level achieves this either consciously or unconsciously with the aid of psychological techniques in order to pull out a peak performance. In endurance sports, performance is also influenced by psychology, although instead of a brief moment of peak concentration or focus, what is required is an underlying, continuous optimization of performance and the willingness to tolerate pain.

Performance reserves in cycling

Psychological training in cycling is still in its infancy and is only used by few cyclists and coaches, especially in track cycling. However, the forms of psychological training are not only interesting for the very top performers for whom this is the only way to improve performance.

Even average racing cyclists and recreational cyclists can achieve incredible results using this type of training, which helps them find an optimal mental attitude and motivation. It also enables tactical and technical movements to be learned more easily and errors to be eliminated. The different relaxation techniques allow the recreational cyclist to cope with stress and help the elite cyclist to attain an optimal state of arousal before the start.

Training world champions

These athletes are very common in cycling; they are cyclists who do very well in training or in performance tests but are unable to reproduce these performances in races, which is one reason why supposedly better cyclists end up losing races. However, the purported strength of these cyclists relates only to their physical fitness; mentally they are a long way from their top form and are unable to perform to their potential when under mental pressure. Interestingly, the cyclists themselves are the cause of this mental pressure, as their good training results lead them and those around them to have high expectations that are never realized.

Not everyone has it

A peak performance, such as winning a tough race or mastering a long ride, involves not only physical factors like endurance and strength, but also intellectual and psychological performance components. These components enable the cyclist to transcend himself, even if this often happens unconsciously. Those who have the correct mental attitude and instinctively do the right thing are lucky, but those who lack this ability will have problems if they do not try to change their mental approach. The training world champion may well be in peak physical shape but is mentally unprepared for racing.

Mental approach

"Anyone who doubts himself can no longer be a successful racing cyclist." "I was thinking about the intensity of the pain that hit me on the mountain and had to drop out." "In every bend in the road I imagined myself slipping! That blocked me, and after every bend I had to close a gap of 5 yards."

These comments show the importance of mental attitude. Mental attitude has a huge influence on both physical and mental motivation and on physical, mental, technical, and tactical performance. Winners are characterized by a high degree of self-confidence, which losers often lack. So the first race victory, the first place, or the first 100-km tour are important steps on the way to sporting self-confidence. Suddenly you are the winner, and this often removes a block that had previously prevented success. However, you should not allow one victory to place you under great pressure to succeed, which may be hard to cope with. Positive thinking and feelings of self-worth and self-confidence are most definitely characteristics of a successful cyclist.

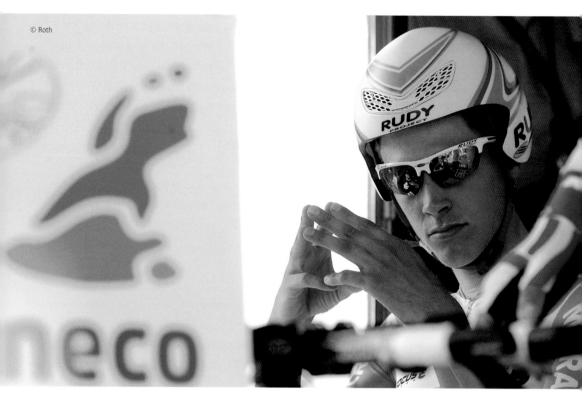

© Roth

Before a time trial, psychological arousal must be optimal.

Winning is all in the head

You must be mentally prepared to give your best, as winning starts in the head and not in the legs. Or to put it negatively: Losing starts in the head. A race or a situation is first lost in the head and only then by the legs. Until you are mentally able to give your all, you will be unable to succeed, unless the race is very easy (an amateur can beat young riders to his heart's content).

An optimal mental approach is the only explanation for athletes achieving results of which they do not seem physically capable.

Flow experience

In such success situations, one is in flow (i.e., mind and body are in harmony). Racing cyclists often describe this flow state retrospectively, saying that they were no longer consciously aware of the extreme challenges (e.g. pain, cold, wind, rain) of a race situation (successful breakaway attempts) or a tour, but just rode relatively loosely and relaxed at a pace that they had never been able to manage before. While people are normally only able to draw on a certain percentage of their absolute performance capacity, in certain mental states it is easier for them to tap these performance reserves. It is mental training that allows the gap between real and absolute performance capacity to be reduced. This capacity that is reserved for extreme situations is called the autonomous protected reserve. Some doping methods give access to part of the protected reserve, which is also what makes them dangerous. The mental strength that paves the way for success is not easy to acquire and needs a good coach. You should improve gradually, race by race and work on yourself. The following sections show what such build-up training could look like.

Look for moderately difficult races

To aid developing mental performance, the races you enter should be neither too easy nor too difficult, but should correspond to your physical and mental shape. A very easy race against weak opponents would lead you to overestimate your ability, while a very hard race would have the opposite effect.

Set realistic goals

Take as much care when setting training goals as when selecting races. If the goal is many years away (e.g., winning a world championship title) and is also unrealistic, you will soon lose sight of it and be aimless again. If a goal is insufficiently challenging, motivation will remain low as will the amount of effort you put into your training and racing. It is advisable for both recreational and elite cyclists to write down their goals, with one relatively far-off but realistic target, such as being selected for a particular team or finishing a 125-mi tour, and smaller, realistic goals, such as winning a particular race or cycling 125 miles in two days. This involves becoming aware of and possibly noting down the obstacles that may stand in the way of achieving these goals and gearing your training toward them (e.g., cornering technique, sprints, climbs, eliminating mental weakness).

Switch off from cycling

To be able to relax mentally and retain your motivation for training and racing, you need to be able to switch off from cycling when training is over. Athletes who think about cycling the whole year day-in, day-out usually have mental blocks and put themselves under too much pressure. You should switch off mentally from cycling, particularly during the transition and preparation phases, but still complete your training program in order to ensure you have sufficient motivation for the racing season.

Motivation

Cyclists need to be highly motivated for training and racing, which becomes all too apparent when you think of a long training ride in bad weather or of the moment when carrying on really hurts and it is just your willpower and motivation that keeps you going. Motivation is greatly influenced by your own evaluation of your performance, and a permanent under- or overestimation prevents success.

This evaluation can be changed by frank discussions with your coach, training partner, parents, or friends. Then use mental training to try to discover and implement available motivation reserves. One simple way of improving motivation is changing the training environment (training camp), taking a break from training (a few days), or practicing other sports in winter. You can also give yourself little rewards for reaching goals.

State of arousal

Many cyclists are too nervous before races and unable to concentrate on the approaching race. The last hour before the race is hectic, and they often forget their drinking bottle or helmet. It is just as difficult for an apathetic cyclist to give of their best. An optimal, average state of arousal is therefore desirable (fig. 7.1).

It is therefore an important goal of mental training to control pre-race emotions and race arousal. Nervous cyclists should work on relaxation techniques, and overly calm ones should boost their motivation.

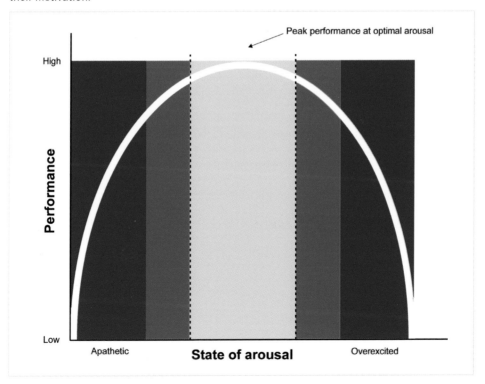

Fig. 7.1: State of arousal. Only a state of optimal arousal allows you to attain peak performance. This graph is greatly simplified as the state of optimal arousal differs from one person to another.

7.2   Relaxation Techniques

You should always use relaxation techniques when you are in a state of emotional tension. Tension caused by anxiety, stress, pressure to succeed, or insecurity is called negative tension, while tension cause by joy, motivation, or self-confidence is referred to as positive tension. Before a race, it is necessary to eliminate the negative tension by means of a relaxation technique, thereby creating an optimal state of arousal. Equally, excessive positive tension can be controlled by a relaxation technique. It is up to the individual to determine their own optimal level of arousal.

Progressive muscle relaxation

Progressive muscle relaxation is a relaxation technique first developed by E. Jacobson in the 1920s, which is highly suitable for sports because it is easy to learn and works well. It involves the isometric contraction (contraction without moving the joints) of individual muscle groups followed by the progressive relaxation of the muscles, which has a psychological effect.

It is best to practice for about 10 minutes each day, for example before going to bed, or in bed if you have trouble going to sleep. Before a race, leave at least 30 minutes between the relaxation phase and the start, otherwise you would be too relaxed. A shortened program can be used to get in the mood for visualization.

Progressive muscular relaxation can be carried out either sitting or lying down, although it is more comfortable and more effective lying down. To start with, it is easier to work with a partner who gives you the relaxation instructions in a calm voice. The techniques should be repeated with each muscle group and are as follows:

1.   Concentrate on the muscles group or the part of the body.

2.   Maximize the contraction of the muscle in question; hold for 8 to 10 seconds.

3.   On a signal, relax for about 30 seconds and concentrate on the area concerned.

Cyclists should start by relaxing the leg muscles, which can be repeated at the end if necessary.

A typical program could be:

1.	left thigh	2.	left lower leg
3.	left foot	4.	right thigh
5.	right lower leg	6.	right foot
9.	left upper arm	10.	left hand and forearm
11.	right upper arm	12.	right hand and forearm
13.	front and back of the neck	14.	face

For example, contract your foot by bending your toes and sole of your foot. Your abs should be hard and firmly contracted and a terrifying grimace etched onto your face. Hold for 8-10 seconds, then relax.

Breathing exercises

Concentrating on your breathing is a quick way of inducing relaxation and also helping you to focus. You need to sit or lie down, close your eyes, and start to breath deliberately. Prolonged exhalation and regular inhalation accelerate the relaxation effect. Your mind should concentrate completely on your breathing. Advanced practitioners can already start visualizing after just a few conscious breaths.

7.3   Mental Training

Visualization

Visualization is an increasingly popular technique that is generally very easy to learn and can help you achieve good results.

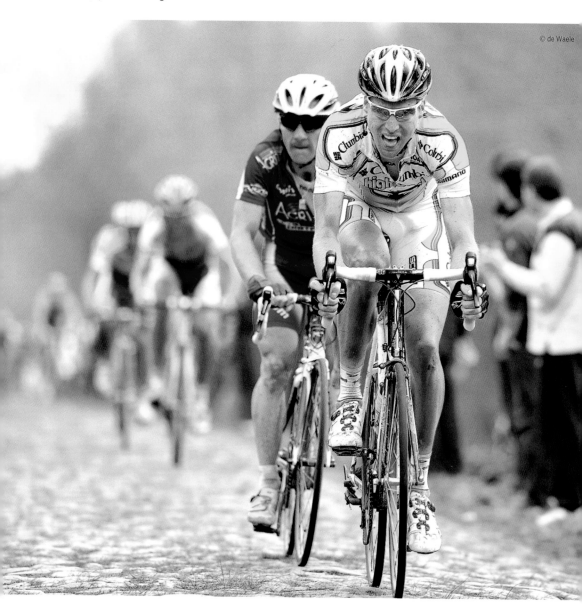

© de Waele

Think in images

Visualization involves freeing yourself from words and thinking in images, which can be supported by noises, smells, and feelings. Allow a movement or action to run before your eyes like film. There is a very close link between movement and the thoughts inside your head, so close that the electrical activity (electromyogram) in the muscle groups normally used in this movement measurably increases just by visualizing the movement. This causes both the muscles and the nervous system to "memorize" the movement, making it easier to put it into practice later on. It is possible to visualize different cycling techniques (e.g., sprinting, cornering, wheelies, braking), an optimal performance, or different emotional target states (e.g., balance, motivation). Likewise after a little practice, tactical situations can also be visualized (e.g., attacking at the right moment, counterattacks, cycling in groups, cycling in the front third of the pack).

It is important to start with simple movements and not to tackle more complicated situations until they have been successfully implemented. Newcomers to mental training should practice for a few minutes as often as possible every day. As with mental training, not all cyclists get the hang of visualization straight away, and it is even possible that some never manage it.

How to do it

Before commencing visualization, put the technique or tactics to be improved in your own words and write them down in detail, about one side of paper. The second step is to read through these notes several times in the days that follow and try to picture the situation in your mind's eye and improve what you have written if necessary. Before starting with the preliminary exercises prior to visualization, take a few moments to relax and calm yourself with the relaxation exercises described previously. When you know your notes by heart, start to imagine the situation with your eyes closed, possibly putting your thoughts into words. It may be helpful to record your notes and play it back on an MP3 player when you first start visualization. The last step is then to visualize the movement, during which you can either observe yourself like the director of a movie (observer's viewpoint) or, better still, by seeing it with your own eyes. The action should take place in the present and never in the past, and always be realistic. Incorrect movement sequences or actions should be avoided in visualization, because they are memorized as incorrect movement patterns. With time and increasing experience of visualization, you will develop your own individual techniques and methods that best meet your personal needs.

Cyclists often reach their mental limits.

Examples of Visualization

Before the race

In the training phase, it is useful to practice mental as well as physical training by visualizing technical, tactical, and mental skills. The pedaling technique, cornering, or climbing are good techniques with which to gain visualization experience.

The day before or directly before a race, visualize the special tactics and mental motivation for the race. Cornering is a skill that can be significantly improved by visualization. More experience is required for tactical visualization.

During the race

On the bike, it is possible to recall an imaginary program without a prior relaxation phase. Brief, tactical instructions (ride at the front, follow a particular cyclist), technical movements (stay on the back wheel when cornering and not braking), and motivational instructions (keep going, give your all, ride loose and light, pedal smoothly) can all be recalled quickly with the aid of the previously practiced images and implemented. These visualizations are often accompanied by silent monologues and silent instructions or self-directed commands.

Imagine motivating images

Cycling, as in other endurance sports, often involves a struggle between mind and body during situations of extreme effort. In situations like these when you are close to breaking point, an individual image helps you to decide the struggle in favor of the mind and makes the task seem easier than it actually is. Whether you choose the image of a beach, a sunny meadow of flowers, a string that is pulling you toward the finishing line, or another positive image is up to you. Imagining something nice—a kind of post-effort reward—can often work wonders and mobilize your hidden final reserves. Also projecting the previously mentioned state of flow, in which everything is light and easy, onto the existing, extremely exhausting situation has been shown to have a performance-enhancing effect.

After the race

After racing or training, the first step is to be aware of any errors committed and then visualize the correct execution, but never remember the error. The imagined movement should always be light and fun. The visualization technique can be performed almost anywhere and especially during breaks from training due to injury.

Example of a visualization program: pedaling technique

1.   Relaxation

Lie on your back, close your eyes, and relax. Now concentrate only on your breathing, which ebbs and flows like waves in the sea. After about one minute, start trying to prolong your exhaled breaths until you automatically start to inhale naturally. This breathing rhythm should also be maintained during the visualization. The wording for the relaxation could go something like this:

I am completely calm and relaxed, completely calm and relaxed. I am peaceful, calm, and relaxed.

My breathing is calm and regular, it ebbs and flows like the waves in the sea.

I now prolong my exhalation, until I start to inhale naturally and automatically.

I am peaceful, calm, and relaxed.

I am now concentrating on my sporting performance.

This text should be repeated two to three times.

2.   Visualization task

The wording for visualizing a smooth pedaling action could go like this. It is important to transfer the words into images and feelings.

I am sitting on the bike and cycling relaxed and fluidly; my legs feel good and I feel good. I pedal, I pull, and I push.

During the whole crank rotation I exercise force onto the pedal.

The approaching climb is easy to cope with, and I ride on smoothly. I pedal, pull, and push. (repeat)

I concentrate on pedaling. I pedal, pull, and push. (repeat)

The bike runs smoothly. In a higher gear I ride smoothly up the mountain, as I feel good.

I pedal, pull, and push. (repeat)

3. Coming to

After visualization, the time for relaxation is over and you open your eyes, stretch, and move.

This, or something like this, is how the wording that is transferred into images in a visualization program should run. Those who have never had anything to do with mental training may at first find all this ridiculous and secretive, but after a few attempts, they will notice that there is more to it than they first thought.

Only consistent practice will allow your visualization technique, and therefore your cycling action, to improve. On the bike, you then only need to recall the image of the smooth pedaling action. A lack of space means that it is unfortunately not possible to go into other movement sequences or tactical situations; visualization programs for other situations can, however, be adapted from this one.

Fear compensation

Many cyclists are always afraid in certain situations; they become blocked which stops them from fulfilling their potential. This fear can be expressed in very different ways and have very different causes. For example, falls can trigger a fear of high cornering speeds or fast descents, a fear so great that the pack is able to pull right away from you.

What is fear?

Fear is a form of mental tension and is very often the psychological escape route from a threatening situation, which could occur or already has occurred (e.g., a fall). As such it is the reflection of the unconscious. As well as the specific fear of falling and its consequences, in mountain biking there are also more complex fears, such as the fear of defeat, victory, or of making a fool of yourself. If you want to do something about your fear, it is important to know and be able to put into words what causes it, as sometimes this is all it takes to make it more manageable. A chat with your coach or a trusted friend can help put things into perspective.

How is fear expressed?

It is difficult for others to diagnose your fear in or before certain situations, for triggers are individual experiences; however there are a few external symptoms that indicate the presence of fear.

- *Physical symptoms:* shaking, stomach problems, pallor, accelerated pulse
- *Motor symptoms:* poor coordination, cramps, mistakes
- *Behavior:* abnormal behavior such as excessive aggression or passivity

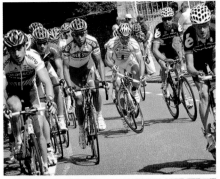

What can you do about fear?

Following are brief presentations of the self-regulating methods that you can do by yourself.

Physical method

First, fear as a state of arousal can be alleviated by physical activity such as an intensive warm-up. Second, the relaxation techniques described next usually really help to get to grips with your fear, as relaxation is the key to controlling fear.

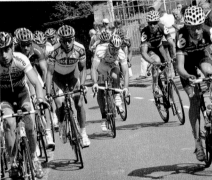

Mental method

In the mental method, the negative thoughts triggered by fear must be reassessed or reinterpreted by trying to think realistically and positively. Reevaluating the importance of a race and seeing it in perspective significantly reduces the pressure and allows you to ride a relaxed race.

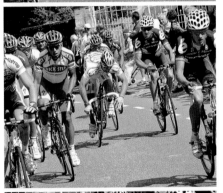

Equipment malfunction: The fear of an equipment malfunction must be eliminated.

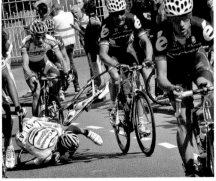

© Roth

As for the very common fear of falling, the greatest success is achieved by visualizing correct, completely safe, and harmonious techniques like cornering, cycling in the peloton, or cycling downhill. However, this should not lead to an increased willingness to take risks, such as in mountain biking downhill races. Incorrect techniques or falls must definitely be excluded from visualization programs and from your thoughts.

7.4   A Pre-Race or Grand Tour Mental Program

The following procedure can be used the day before a race or on race day to prepare mentally for the coming performance. Leave a gap of at least 30 minutes between the end of the routine and the start of the race (ideally at home before leaving for the race). Seek out a comfortable place where you can be undisturbed for about 20 minutes and can sit down or, even better, lie down. Your legs should lie loosely next to each other without touching, and your feet should fall slightly to the side.

1.   **Progressive muscle relaxation**

With your eyes closed, first relax your body using your own or the muscle relaxation program provided here, paying particular attention to your legs.

2.   **Positive thinking**

Now move mentally to a beautiful place that suggests peace, safety, and relaxation; it can be a meadow, a beach, the forest, or similar. Your mind should now stay in this place and concentrate only on positive thoughts.

3.   **Visualization**

The third step, taken after you have successfully achieved physical and mental relaxation, is to visualize the coming race or tour. This involves imagining you are on the course and implementing your positive, successful tactics. Anticipated difficulties (e.g., climbs) are easily taken in stride. You try to create a positive, performance-affirming attitude toward the coming race, which should be enjoyable.

4.   **Coming to**

Once you have visualized a successful end to the race (whatever form that may take), you should snap out of the relaxation by shaking out and stretching. On race day, you should now focus on starting your warm-up. The evening before a race you don't need to return to reality so abruptly, especially if you are going to bed immediately afterward.

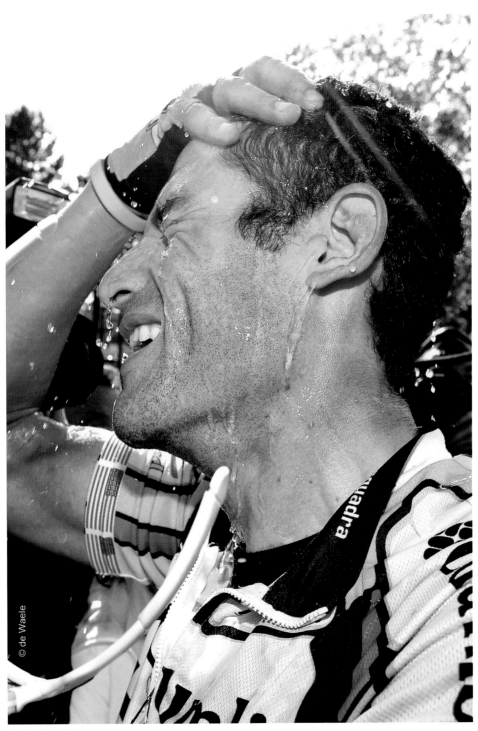

© de Waele

Total exhaustion

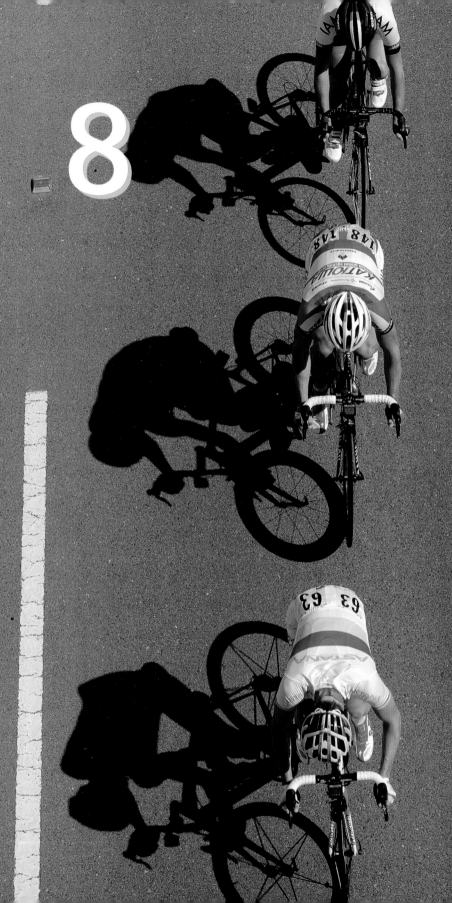

8   Cycling Technique

8.1   The Correct Cycling Position

There is a limit to how much a person on a racing bike can adapt to the machine. For man and bicycle to be in perfect harmony, the bike must be adjusted to fit the rider and not vice versa. It is therefore very important to choose the correct frame size and to adjust the bike correctly. In the cycling scene, there are a multitude of tips and formulae for finding the correct cycling position, many of them based on the experiences of racing cyclists, and they seem to work quite well. As well as these rules of thumb, computer programs have been developed in recent years that can calculate the optimal position based on scientific research. The truth regarding the perfect sitting position lies, as it so often does, somewhere in between the two. The combination of rule of thumb, scientific methods, and, above all, experience, helps cyclists find the right position for them, which does not hurt and allows them to fully develop their performance potential.

The first task of newcomers to cycling or those with a new bike must be to set up their bike correctly. There are a few rules to be observed, though sometimes even these rules need to be broken in order to find the best position for you. Orthopedic problems like back pain (lumbar area) or knee problems require adapted sitting positions that will be explored in more detail next.

Once you have found your position, it is advisable to make a note of the measurements so that a new or borrowed bike can quickly be tailored to your body and to avoid time-consuming experimenting and possible aches and pains in the musculoskeletal system.

Setting the right position in seven steps
The different steps in the process of setting the correct position must be carried out in the right order as they are interdependent. A typical procedure is described next.

1.   Saddle height

The saddle height is the first and most important adjustment that must be made to the bike. Start by choosing a frame that is suitable for your body height, as one that is too big or too small will make adjustments very difficult. So if you start with the right frame size, the only way of regulating the saddle height is by adjusting the seat post.

Table 8.1: Overview of seating adjustment

Sequence	Measurement	Tool	Aids
1	Saddle height	Allen key 4, 5, or 6 mm	Wall or partner, book, measuring tape, calculator
2	Saddle angle	Allen key 5 or 6 mm	Spirit level
3	Saddle position	Allen key 5 or 6 mm	Plumb line
4	Pedal adjustment	Allen key 4 mm	Possible pedal tool or helper
5	Handlebar height	Allen key 4 or 5 mm	Helper, different stems
6	Seating length	Allen key 4 or 5 mm	Helper, different stems
7	Crank length	Allen key 5 or 10 mm	

In bikes with old-fashioned clip pedals there is a way of adjusting the saddle height that cannot be used very accurately in bikes with safety pedals due their different structure, although it does give an approximate guide.

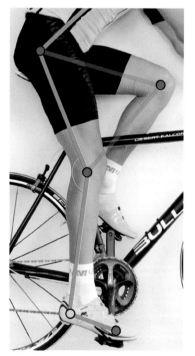

Fig. 8.1: Saddle height

Sit on the bike and support yourself against a wall. With your heels placed on the bottom of the pedals, straighten your legs as you pedal backward, without sliding about in the saddle and making sure you extend your knees fully. If your shoes are locked in the pedals, your leg extension at the lower pedal position should be 140 to 155 degrees. Your legs are therefore stretched quite wide at the knee joint, but don't push your heel down or raise it.

The angle to be measured is that between the lateral malleolus, the middle of the knee slightly above the head of the fibula and the large trochanter, a bump that can be felt in the femur at hip level.

Individual adjustments

Different saddle heights are preferred depending on the discipline and type of cyclist; a low frequency cyclist, like many time trialists or climbers, have a rather high saddle so that they can straighten their legs as much as possible, generating high torque, while a points racer or criterium specialist would tend to prefer a lower saddle to allow him to maintain a high cadence over long periods of time and to react better to changes of speed.

So, to summarize, a lower saddle height and therefore low knee extension is advantageous at high cadences, while a higher saddle works better at lower cadences with correspondingly higher power. Road cyclists will choose a medium height to enable them to cope with widely differing types of effort.

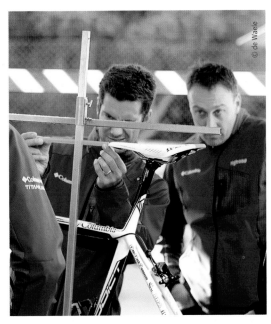

Hügi method

This formula has proved to be an effective way of determining this medium position, which is used to set the saddle height accurately. The first step is to measure the leg length by standing against a wall in bare feet with the feet together and with the aid of the back of a book that is pushed into the crotch

If you have several bikes, the position must be exactly the same for them all.

(perpendicular to the wall). Make a mark on the wall and then measure it. This value is then multiplied by 0.885 to arrive at the saddle height (center of the crank to the top of the saddle). The result is a very low sitting position. If you would like to sit higher, you can increase the factor to 0.895. This does not take into account the pedal system, the thickness of the soles of the shoes, and the crank length of the cycling shoes.

Feel matters

Regardless of all these formulae and suggestions, how you feel on your bike should be your main guide when it comes to adjusting saddle height. Theoretical formula cannot take into account all your individual prerequisites and for this reason should just be used as a guide.

If your bike has clipless pedals, you should follow the manufacturer's instructions for adjusting the saddle height if they are provided. When purchasing new shoes and before fitting a new pedal system, you should measure the distance from the inner sole of the shoe (above the axis) to the top edge of the saddle (with the crank parallel to the saddle tube) in order to be able to set the same saddle height for the new shoes or pedals.

Recreational cyclists tend to position their saddles too low, which completely stops them from developing maximum power and also puts too much strain on the knees. New saddles lose height after being used for a certain amount of time as they become flattened, making it necessary to readjust the saddle height raising it by a fraction of an inch. If you suffer from knee problems, depending on the type of complaint or injury, the saddle height will also need to be either lowered or raised, as described in more detail in chapter 6.

Raise the saddle gradually

If you notice that the saddle height is actually too low, as a frequent cyclist you should raise it gradually, at a rate of around a quarter of an inch every two weeks, in order to prevent joint pain. Even occasional cyclists should never raise the saddle dramatically from one day to the next.

2. Saddle angle

As well as the height of the saddle, the tilt must also be adjusted. A racing saddle will be set exactly horizontal to the ground as this ensures the best pressure distribution thus helping to prevent saddle sores and pressure points. If the saddle points downward, the pressure on the arms is too high and you will constantly be slipping forward. An upward-pointing saddle may well stop you slipping forward but it will put too much pressure on the urethra, which can be very painful (chapter 6). On top of that, the hips are tilted to the rear by this saddle position so that the joints in the lumbar spine are put under greater strain, and this may lead to pain and, at worst, even deteriorations in the vertebral body over several years. The saddle angle is best checked using a spirit level.

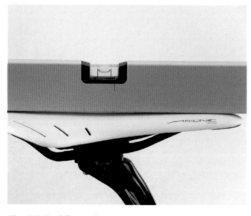

Fig. 8.2: Saddle angle

3. Saddle position

Saddle position means the position of the saddle on the seat post; the saddle can be shifted several inches backward and forward on its frame. When setting the saddle position, it is already parallel to the ground, and the cyclist must just sit normally on it. The pedal plates must also already be adjusted. Starting from a mid-position of the saddle, you can start the fine-tuning. A plumb line hanging from the saddle tip should cut about one to three inches behind the center of the bottom bracket of the chain stay. Cyclists with very long or short thighs will obviously deviate from this position.

However, when making these adjustments you must bear in mind the regulations of the UCI, which stipulate a minimum setback distance of 2 inches. Only very short cyclists with special permission may sit farther forward. This rule was introduced in connection with the aerodynamic sitting position in hour world records and in track disciplines. It is reported that checks are only occasionally carried out in time trials.

Where the saddle is positioned within this area is determined as follows: With crank position, drop a plumb line from the front of the knee through the pedal axis. If it doesn't touch the pedal axis, the saddle must be moved so that the plumb line at least falls very near the axis. Road-racing cyclists prefer a position behind the pedal axis (0.2 in), in which they sit farther back making it easier to ride with high gears.

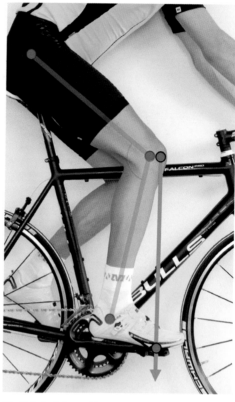

Fig. 8.3: Saddle position

4.   Pedal adjustment

If you want to avoid joint damage in the future to your knees, feet, and hips, your cleats must be adjusted very carefully. Often, incorrectly set up cleats that only cause very slight discomfort when pedaling are left as they are out of laziness. Over the course of a year, this can lead to knee damage. So even if pedaling is only slightly uncomfortable following pedal adjustment, the pedals must be moved very carefully until they feel right.

The foot is normally placed in the pedals parallel to the crank. In a longitudinal direction, the pedals are set up so that the joint at the base of the big toe (metatarsophalangeal joint) sits exactly over the center of the pedal axis, as this is the only way to ensure an effective transfer of power, because the force passes through the ball of the foot as it does in running. A real help in setting up the pedals is that the joint cavity (bony growth on the inside of the big toe) can be felt through the shoe and then pushed above the middle of the pedal axis. Many pedal manufacturers provide good set-up aids in the form of templates or brochures, without which it is very difficult to achieve an optimal adjustment of the sometimes very complicated pedal system. A few pedal systems, such as those manufactured by TIME, only require pedals to be set up longways, and no lateral adjustment is required due to a sideways room for a maneuverability of 5 degrees (it is very useful to have someone to help you in all position adjustments).

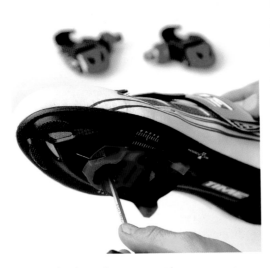

Fig. 8.4: The cleat adjustment must be very accurate.

After making the longitudinal adjustments, the angle to the crank must be set. Starting from the parallel position that is identical on both sides, the heel or the whole foot can be moved very gradually until it is in the right place. It is possible for each side to be set up differently. Then test it out by pedaling backward or forward on the roller. This adjustment works best with hand-tightened screws that allow the foot to twist when the cleats are clipped in. Once you find the position, pull out the shoe hanging on the pedal without turning the cleat and mark the cleat position clearly on the sole of the shoe with a felt-tipped pen. Upon release, the plate turns, but with the aid of the marking, it can be repositioned and tightened.

5. Handlebar height

The handlebar height is limited by the length of the steering tube. The handlebar height should be set so that the difference in height between the top edge of the saddle and that of the handlebar is a maximum of 2.5 to 3 inches. The occasional cyclist's saddle and handlebar will both be set at roughly the same height. Greater differences put strain on the spine and, particularly in young riders, can cause degenerative changes in the spine. The lumbar and thoracic areas of the spine are excessively curved, and the cervical spine is overextended due to the low grip position. If you have very long arms, though, a greater height difference is sometimes necessary.

However, if you still feel pain in the area of the lumbar or cervical spine, you must change your position. Height differences of more than 4 or 5 inches are not uncommon, and even 8 inches is not unheard of. If you already have back problems (e.g. slipped disc) or pain, there should be as little difference as possible between the height of your handlebar and saddle.

If you have a new bike, do not shorten the steering tube until you are sure of the handlebar height after plenty of test rides. Height can only be gained by a shorter and slightly upward-pointing stem. Frames with high set head tubes also make for a comfortable position. If the handlebar is set lower, you just need to remove the spacer under the stem and put it on top. Everything will then be ok and the steering tube around the area (spacer above the stem) can be shortened.

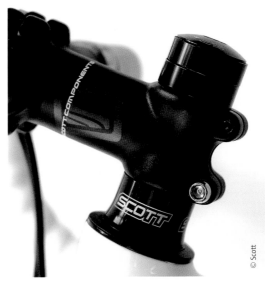

© Scott

Fig. 8.5: Spacer on top

The muscle tensions felt by newcomers to cycling or experienced cyclists at the start of the season are usually short-lived and disappear with improved flexibility and performance capacity of the back muscles.

© Scott

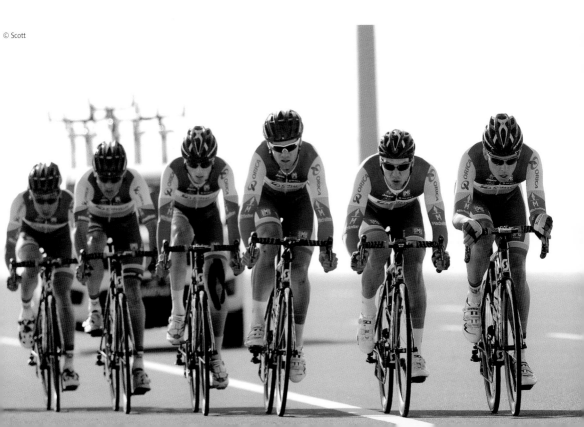

6. Seating length, or fore–aft saddle position

This is the distance from the tip of the saddle to the center of the handlebar. It is determined by the top tube length of the frame, the stem length, and the saddle position. If you buy a frame off the shelf, it will have a standard top tube length corresponding to the frame height, and if you buy a made-to-measure bike you will have limited input regarding the length of the top tube.

In general, frames should be as small and therefore as short as possible, and the stem should be as long as possible. A 2.5- to 3-inch longer stem on a big frame would be out of place, as a considerably smaller frame could be selected. The saddle position should, if possible, not be used to regulate the fore–aft seat position, as it will already have been adjusted to suit your leg length. So the seating length can only be adjusted by changing the stem length. The handlebar shape also affects the fore–aft saddle position, particularly when the hands are on the hoods and on the drops when the difference between a short or long and deep handlebar can amount to a matter of inches. The best way to do it is to hold the curves of the handlebar next to each other at the specialist store and measure the depth of the handlebar.

Feel is the most important factor when adjusting the fore–aft saddle position, as you must feel comfortable on your bike.

How long?
There is a simple way of checking whether you have the correct fore–aft position, although this is just a rule of thumb and only gives an approximate value.

a. Leaning against a wall or supported by a partner, place your hands on the drops, gripping them, and bring a crank into a parallel position to the down tube. In this position, elbows and knees should only be inches away from each other.

b. Another rule of thumb states that in deep handlebar positions (holding the drops) with slightly bent elbows, the front wheel hub should be covered by the upper handle bar. The position should neither be too stretched and flat nor too upright. The hoods grip and drops grip must both be comfortable over long distances without the back complaining. Once the bike is completely set up, the newcomer to cycling may initially find the position uncomfortable and very stretched out, but this sensation should disappear after the first 600 miles, as the body very quickly gets used to this new situation.

7. Crank length

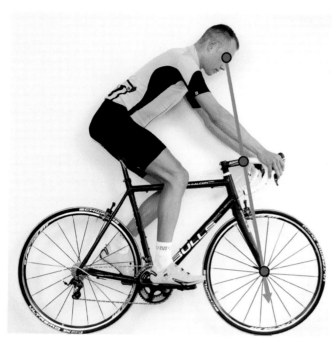

Fig. 8.6: Fore–aft saddle position

Racing cranks are manufactured in lengths of 165 to 180 mm. The normal length is 170 mm, although this varies according to discipline and body size. Time trial and mountain cyclists prefer a slightly longer crank (175 mm), while circuit and track cyclists use shorter cranks (170 mm, 165 mm on the track). It would be difficult to provide rules stating which crank length should be used for which leg length or body height. The short crank allows for higher cadence, while the long crank ensures a better power transfer (longer lever), naturally at the expense of cadence and corner angle. With slightly shorter cranks, a criterium specialist can continue pedaling round corners, where long cranks would require him to stop pedaling. Every racing cyclist swears by his optimal crank length. However, it is wise for children to use shorter cranks (165 mm) and very tall cyclists to use long cranks (175-180 mm). Nevertheless, the importance of crank length should not be overestimated. There is certainly no point in beginners changing cranks just to be able to pedal with an inch longer crank. The possible benefit in no way justifies the cost. Amazingly, the subject of crank length is accorded no importance at all, and all cyclists, regardless of their height, ride with 175 mm cranks and use the same length on their road bikes.

Bike fit card

Once you have found your ideal position, it is worth preparing a measuring card with all the important set-up measurements to help you set up a new bike quickly. The following measurements should be noted:

1. Frame height (center of the bottom bracket to top edge of the seat tube)

2. Seat height (center of the bottom bracket to top edge of the saddle)

3. Frame length (center of the head tube to center of the seat tube)

4. Fore–aft saddle position (saddle tip to center of the handlebars)

5. Stem length (INBUS center to center of the head tube)

6. Saddle rise (vertical difference between saddle and handlebar height)

7. Seat set-back (horizontal distance between the tip of the saddle and the center of the bottom bracket)

8. Crank length (center of the bottom bracket to center of the pedal axis)

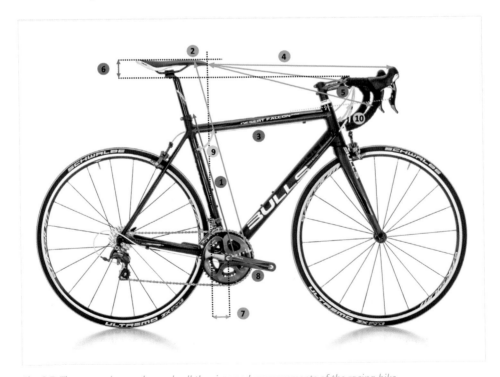

Fig. 8.7: The measuring card records all the sizes and measurements of the racing bike.

9.   Seat tube angle

10. Head tube angle

11. Handlebar reach and drop

12. Bottom bracket width and pedal distance

8.2   Smooth Pedal Action

A smooth pedal action is defined as an even exertion of power on the pedal throughout the whole pedaling cycle. However, the even exertion of power in every movement phase is only theoretically possible due to the difference in strength between the muscle groups of the leg (quadriceps and hamstrings). The quadriceps always undertake most of the forward propulsion work. The smooth pedal action is what separates the racing cyclist from the recreational cyclist. Because the foot is attached to the pedal on a racing bike, it is not only possible to pedal—exert power downwards—but also to push and pull, which the recreational cyclist is unable to do with his conventional pedals.

The term pedaling cycle is a little misleading and does not describe the actual situation; crank cycle or crank rotation cycle would be more neutral terms.

Use your hamstrings

If you only pedal downward, you are ignoring an important muscle group in the leg, the hamstrings. You should aim to use as many leg and hip muscle groups as possible in order to take some pressure off the hardworking quadriceps in your efforts to drive yourself forward. A lot of scientific research has shown that only a very few cyclists are able to achieve a smooth pedal action. Pedaling technique must be taught from a young age and even at high performance level, your program should include regular pedaling technique training.

Pedaling

The pedaling technique should be fluid, smooth, and correct, keeping the legs and especially the knees close to the frame. The upper body and head should be kept as still as possible so as to avoid wasting energy in unnecessary muscle movements. The upper body should only move when sprinting or in tough mountain passages. The power for the pedaling cycle comes mainly from the leg muscles and cannot be reinforced by rocking the head or torso. However, torso and arm muscles are used in pedaling in that they help to stabilize the body during the one-sided forward-propulsion downward action of each leg. The hand, arm, shoulder, abdomen, and back form a muscle sling anchored in the torso and hips, which alternates rhythmically from side to side. The function of this muscle sling becomes clear when you ride out of the saddle, when the simultaneous arm and other structures involved constitute the resistance to the straightening action of the leg. This muscle sling has to work especially hard when you cycle in high gears.

During the era of the former GDR (German Democratic Republic), experiments were carried out with additional resistance in the form of a rope that tied the upper body to the frame and was intended to enable better power development as it took the pressure off the supporting muscles.

Core stability training

The need for general athletic training that develops strong but not bulky arm and torso muscles is obvious as far as the supporting and resisting functions are concerned. Leg strength measurements in athletes have shown that it is rare for both legs to be equally strong. Likewise, there are very few cyclists who are able to generate the same amount of propulsive power with both legs, although this is a prerequisite for a perfect, smooth pedaling action and for the avoidance of orthopedic problems. If you are diagnosed with a muscular imbalance (difference in strength between the legs or agonist and antagonist muscles), you should follow a targeted strength program supervised by a physical therapist in order to balance out the difference.

Crank cycle in eight sectors

The **crank cycle** can easily be divided into three different parts:

1. The push-down phase in which the quads push the pedal down.

2. The pull-up phase, which runs from the bottom dead center to just before the top dead center and is carried out by the hip and knee flexors.

3. The push-forward phase, in which the foot is pushed forward at the top dead center.

There is some overlap in the start and finish of these three phases. A more exact breakdown is shown in figure 8.8, in which the cycle is divided into eight sectors of 45 degrees each.

First Sector

In the first sector of the cycle, the pedaling or push-down phase starts at about 10 degrees. At the end of this sector, the push-forward phase starts.

Second and Third Sectors

In these two sectors, the greatest pedaling power is developed by the extensor muscles in the

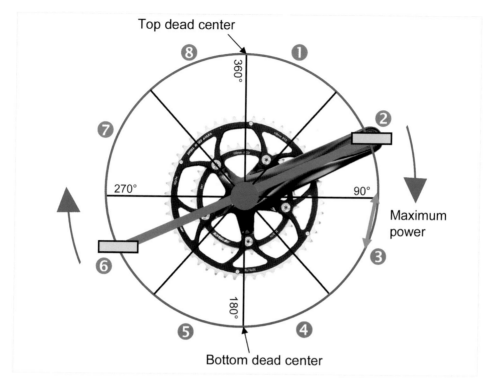

Fig. 8.8: Pedaling cycle divided into sectors

leg (hamstrings, glutes, calf muscles), which, expressed as a percentage, represent the majority of the propulsion power. Maximum power is usually exerted (depending on the cyclist) between 90 and 110 degrees.

Fourth Sector

The pull-up phase starts here in the muscles, even before the pedaling phase has finished and is still generating a great deal of power.

Fifth Sector

Between the fourth and fifth sectors, at 180 degrees, lies the **bottom dead** center of the crank rotation cycle. Characteristic of both transition points is that here, at least theoretically, only the crank can be shortened or extended. A rotation is not possible. The lower transition point must be overcome by the early use of the quadriceps (i.e., an early introduction of the pull-up phase with momentum). The other leg assists with a pronounced push-forward phase at the top dead center. In the fifth section, from about 200 degrees, the pedal can be pulled back and up with greater power due to the better lever ratio.

Sixth and Seventh Sections

In the sixth and seventh sections, the main work is done in the pulling phase; hip flexors, hamstrings, and shin muscles pull the pedal back and up.

Eighth Section

The push-forward phase starts in the eighth section at around 320 degrees. The top dead center of the crank rotation cycle is passed through with the aid of the quadriceps muscle.

On a normal bike, the conventional design of the pedals mean that no pulling force is exerted on them. The weight of the leg is only raised by the pedaling power of the other leg, which is a considerable waste of energy. For the pedaling action to be efficient, the transitions between the push-down, pull-up, and push-forward phases must be as smooth as possible and complement each other cyclically on both crank arms.

Foot position

The position of the foot during the crank rotation cycle varies depending on the cadence.

At **low cadences** (up to 85 rpm), particular attention can be paid to each phase. Low cadences are usually combined with a high to very high power exertion at high intensities. In the push-forward and pull-up phases, the slow movement means that more power can be exerted onto the pedals than at high cadences. During the push-down phase, the heel is lowered and the toes are slightly raised, while during the pull-up phase, the toes point right down.

Medium cadences (from 85-105 rpm) require less ankle work, which is reflected in a more or less horizontal foot position. The foot movements mentioned in the previous section are still made, but with a reduced range of motion.

High cadences (over 105 rpm) place high motor demands on the coordination of the participating muscles. High speeds mean that there is less time for muscle contraction, and the heels must therefore be raised during the entire crank rotation cycle. The range of motion during the pedaling action is reduced, and the ankle is almost rigidly fixed in this position.

Scientific studies have shown that trained cyclists prefer a flatter foot position compared to occasional cyclists. They lower their heels in the push phase so that they are below the toes, while occasional cyclists prefer a foot position in which the heel is slightly raised.

Pedaling technique training

A smooth pedaling action, or at least an approximation of it, is essential at high performance level. There are many ways of working on this.

One-Leg Training

In order to experience what it actually means to exert a constant force on the pedals, try pedaling with only one leg for 110 yards or 50 revolutions. You need to concentrate on the pull-up, push-forward, and push-down phases if you want to move forward. Three repetitions per leg of this little exercise can be included in every workout.

Slow and Deliberate

High gears, as in strength endurance training, combined with low cadences allow you to deliberately coordinate and vary each phase of the cycle, making you more aware of all phases of the pedal cycle.

Fixed-Gear Bikes

High cadences also train a smooth pedaling action as they require a pull-up phase for an economical pedaling style. In winter training, cycling with fixed gears has proven to be a good way of practicing this as there is no freewheel mechanism and you cannot stop pedaling. To be able to move forward on a fixed-gear bike, the muscles must pedal more or less constantly. Choose gear ratios of 42/39 x 15-20 and in the first part of the preparation phase ride about 300 to 700 mi with fixed gears on roads that are as flat as possible. The lower the gear ratio, the greater the benefit of fixed-gear training. Training speed is irrelevant.

There are two other ways of training a smooth pedaling action which do not focus on the movement itself on the legs, but where the movement is conceived and planned in the head. First, in a kind of dry run training, in your lounge, or in indoor training, imagine executing a perfect, smooth pedaling action.

This is called visualization (described in more detail in chapter 7), and it eventually leads to an improvement in technique in practice.

Reminder Note

Alternatively, you can write a little note saying: *Smooth pedaling action: push forward, push down, pull up, especially pull back and push up.* Then stick this note to the bike handlebar or stem as a constant reminder of the correct movement during training.

When to train pedaling technique?

Technique practice can be added to shorter basic or compensatory training sessions, and this can include other techniques such as jumps or cornering. The hard part of the smooth pedaling action is not pushing down but pushing forward and pulling, hence the importance of these words on the note to make you focus on the correct movements. While this may seem a little exaggerated, it really does help when it comes to learning and improving the smooth pedaling action. Of course you can also focus on pushing forward and pulling up without the visual reminder of this note.

8.3 Grip Positions on the Handlebar

The curved shape of racing handlebars allows for many different grip positions. Depending on the situation, you can hold the handlebars down on the drops, on the hoods (brakes), or relaxed on the top bar.

Top bar

Whether you are cycling in a group or training alone, the top bar grip is the ideal position for a relaxed posture in which you can ride comfortably for hours. The hands can grip in different places right along the top of the bar to the brake levers (hoods). This position is not suitable for fast cycling in races though, as it is not aerodynamically sound and you cannot use the brakes. Neither is it advisable when cycling out of the saddle, as it is very unstable.

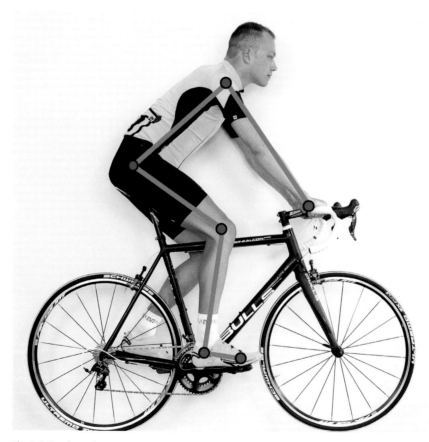

Fig. 8.9: Top bar grip

Hoods grip

Holding the hoods is a grip that is also very popular for racing. It is more aerodynamic than the top bar grip and, above all, safer, as the brakes can be accessed from this position and difficult handlebar maneuvers can be carried out. As your back is less flat than in the drops grip, you are able to get a better overview of the traffic or racing situation, and in the mountain and when sprinting, the hoods grip allows powerful control of the handlebars. The hoods grip and the top bar grip are therefore ideal for training.

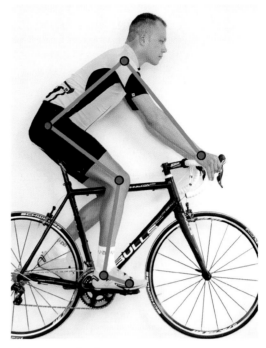

Fig. 8.10: Hoods grip

Drops grip

In racing and in fast sections, the drops grip is the ideal position as it is very aerodynamic. In training, it is much too uncomfortable to be used in long rides. However, the back muscles must get used to the low position. The handlebar is held at the top, in the middle, or at the end of the drops. In very fast sections, you need to flatten your back completely against the frame so that the forearms are parallel with the road. This position is also possible using the hoods grip. If the traffic situation becomes hard to monitor or dangerous, the hooks grip with the fingers on the brakes is the safest grip as it allows optimal steering and braking.

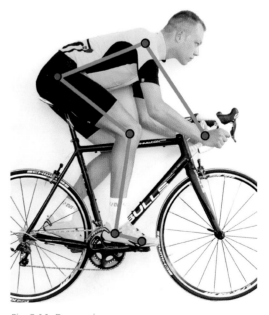

Fig. 8.11: Drops grip

8.4   Climbing Position

Climbing requires a special technique in order to conquer the climb most efficiently. The low speed makes an aerodynamic sitting position irrelevant. Normally, the preference is for a wide top bar grip with relaxed back and shoulders that hinders breathing as little as possible. Whether you use the hoods grip to climb in a sitting position is up to you, because sometimes it makes cyclists feel over-extended and that their breathing is impeded. When riding out of the saddle, though, the hoods grip is ideal. The drops grip is only used in climbing for break-away attempts and on flat sections.

On steep, long climbs, it makes sense to alternate between cycling in and out of the saddle, because then the muscle groups used are also alternated. Less steep climbs at an even pace should mainly be tackled in a sitting position, because riding out of the saddle is less energy efficient than the sitting position.

If you do ride in the sitting position, your own rhythm and choice of gear ratio are very important, so that a fluid, high-cadence style has proven to be more efficient with a low gear ratio than an energetic "stamping" style with a high gear ratio. Although this does depend what kind of cyclist you are.

Riding out of the saddle

Riding out of the saddle is a demanding technique and requires a lot of practice for beginners. It is mainly used for accelerating and very steep sections. It involves shifting the bodyweight over the almost straightened legs while the bike is tilted from side to side by the pulling action of the arms. The key is to avoid the body swaying back and forth; it is the bike that should be tilted under the body. In the process, the bodyweight participates fully in the downward movement of the crank, supported by the pushing of the arm on the same side of the body and the pulling of the arm on the opposite side. If a lot of power is exerted on the pedals (final sprints, climbs), the arms alternately pull and push on the handlebar, while at low pedaling power and higher cadence, the arm action is limited to a pushing down of the opposite arm.

Zig-zagging

The pulling and pushing action of the arms should not cause unnecessary movements of the handlebar that make the bike move in a zig-zag fashion. It is very common to see this in sprints, particularly among young cyclists. It is inefficient due to the longer distance traveled but looks impressive. In sprints and climbs, all your strength must be used to move forward.

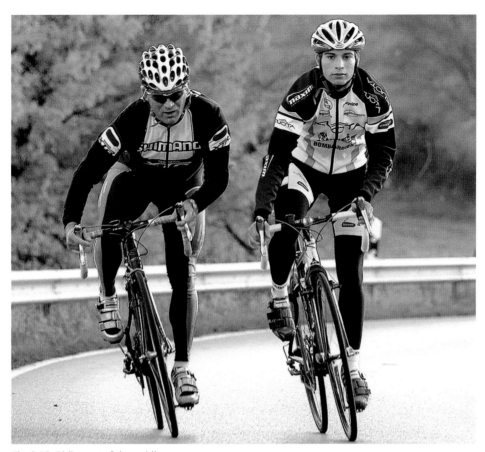

Fig. 8.12: Riding out of the saddle

Descent position

Adopt an aerodynamic position when cycling downhill in order to reach the bottom with as little air resistance as possible. The most diverse and sometimes very daring and dangerous positions can be observed; however, a position with horizontal cranks, knees close to the frame, narrow arm position, and bent over upper body is sufficient in most cases and still allows you keep an eye on and react quickly to the situation. It still allows you to rise out of the saddle a little and if necessary hold one arm behind your back.

If you prefer a position in which your nose almost touches the front wheel, you must pull your head back to be able to see where you are going. In descents, the tempo is usually so high that you are no longer able to pedal. To allow your legs to recover slightly, keep pedaling gently, shake out your muscles occasionally, and stretch a little. Extremely aerodynamic positions constitute hard static work for the leg muscles.

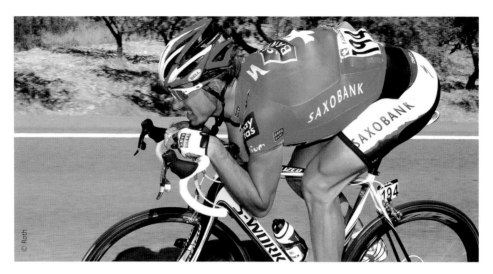

Fig. 8.13: Descent – Fabian Cancellara in a safe aero position

Descents require a great deal of concentration, and particularly in races, dangerous situations can arise, hence the need for concentration. When your strength allows, during the climb you should move forward to the first third so that in the ensuing descent you are not left by the wayside. It is best to begin a descent near the front of the pack.

8.5   Correct Braking Technique

Braking causes the circumferential speed of the wheels to slow down due to the friction of the brake linings on the wheel rims, and the kinetic energy is almost completely converted into heat by friction. On long descents, strong braking can cause the tire temperature to climb so dramatically that the tire glue of tubular tires melts and the tires eventually pop out of the rims or the valve bursts. This is why you should not brake continuously, but intermittently before corners.

Effective front wheel brake
Front and rear brakes are not equally strong: The front brake is up to a third more effective than the rear brake, because in the braking process, the main load shifts to the front wheel and therefore the traction of the front wheel on the road increases significantly. Because of the lower traction, the rear wheel blocks much more quickly than the front wheel.

It is also important to learn to brake gradually so that the wheels don't block, making you slip or get catapulted over the handlebars. You should also regularly practice full braking so that you can react correctly in a dangerous situation in a race or in traffic. Basically, you should brake with both levers and aim for a gradual braking process. If you suddenly need to brake sharply, it is advisable to pull the brake lever once very sharply and then let it go slightly and finally brake gradually. Pulling on the brakes as hard as possible without relaxing your grip has fatal consequences. However this is what people tend to do in an emergency if they are not familiar with their braking system. Intermittent braking (as done when driving a car) is completely unsuitable for use in cycling, as in a group it would endanger the riders behind you. As there is no technical solution for the blocking of the wheels on a racing bike, it is up to the cyclist to take responsibility for this by means of a sophisticated braking technique and a lot of experience.

Emergency stop

In an emergency stop, when you brake suddenly before a corner or in a descent, your body's center of gravity is shifted backward as your arms are extended and your bottom is pushed back over the saddle. Emergency braking is worse in the rain than on dry tires, hence the importance of braking well before a corner in order to break down the film of water on the tires so that the brake pads can do their job. In descents or in city traffic, you should therefore keep light pressure on the brake levers but with no noticeable braking effect.

8.6   Correct Cornering Technique

The correct cornering technique is crucial for safe cycling in street traffic and also to be able to participate successfully in races. Beginners find it particularly difficult, and this often puts them in unnecessarily dangerous situations. An incorrect cornering technique is often the reason why beginners quickly drop off the pace in races. Young cyclists in particular must pay great attention to learning the correct cornering technique as part of cycling-specific technique and skills training.

Cornering physics

When you take a corner, centrifugal force is exerted on you and your bike. Centrifugal force pulls the cyclist out of the corner and is determined by the joint mass of the cyclist and bike, the cornering speed, and the corner radius. In simplified terms, this means that the heavier the

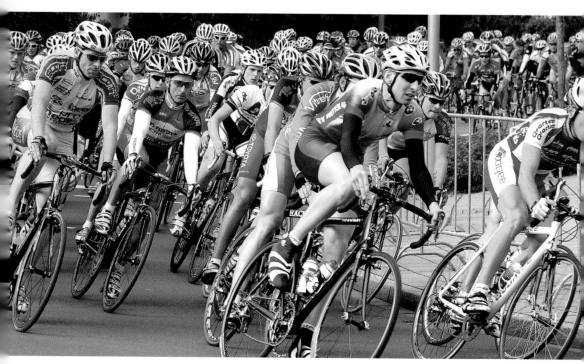

The peloton taking a corner

cyclist and bike, the higher the speed and the narrower the corner, the greater the centrifugal force, and the more difficult it is to negotiate the corner successfully, as the grip of the tires starts to be pushed to the limit. As both the mass and corner radius are fixed values, the centrifugal force can only be kept in check by a reduction in speed. Greatly simplified, if the centrifugal force exceeds the tire grip, the cyclist will fall from his bike.

Cornering tips

Speed must be reduced before the corner to reduce the likelihood of slipping on an unchanged road surface, and only experience will teach you to what extent you need to do this. The braking process should basically be completed before the corner so that you just need to make small corrections as you take the corner. In races and descents, the drops grip is the best position for negotiating corners safely, because it keeps the body's center of gravity low, increasing your stability. The higher the speed around the corner, the greater the lean on the part of bike and cyclist. You should try to keep in the same plane as the bike so that both lean equally into the corner. The knees should be close to the frame; the inside knee may be angled in emergencies in order to shift more weight toward the center of rotation without having to lean more into the corner. The inside pedal is brought round to the top position to prevent it from scraping on the ground. The outer leg is extended and exerts pressure on the outer pedal, which stabilizes the cornering process.

Ideal line

If you would like to carry on pedaling around corners (e.g., in criteriums), you need a great deal of experiences and flat pedals that allow a flatter lean angle. The corner is taken along what is called the ideal line—it is approached as wide as possible. You then cut in at the apex and ride out of it as wide as possible. By cutting the corner, you increase (from a physical point of view) the curve radius at the apex of the curve, thereby reducing the centrifugal force. This technique is of course impossible in normal road traffic conditions and should only be used in completely cordoned off race courses, as in road races, obstacles can pop up at corners which are almost impossible to avoid. In these cases, it is advisable to keep a little margin of safety to allow last-minute deviations if necessary.

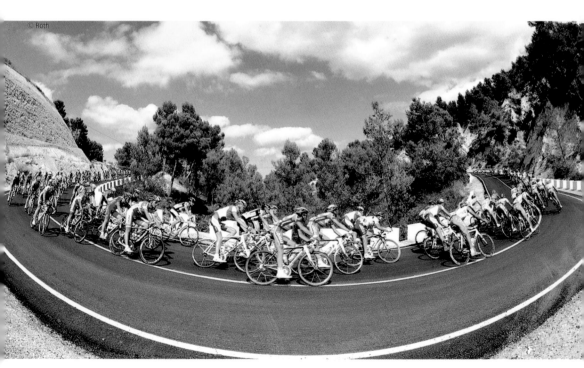

Fig. 8.14: Ideal line: approach wide – cut in – exit wide

Cornering in the peloton

In races, at high speeds it is best to ride on the inside, leaving about 1.5 feet leeway from the curb for other cyclists who are struggling; inside is better because here the danger of getting tangled up with cyclists skidding outward in a fall is significantly lower. It is better to take a corner near the front of the peloton that is cornering without braking hard. In the middle or the rear of the peloton, cyclists usually brake hard as they corner which means that they must pedal harder afterward to make up lost ground.

Hazards around the corner

If you suddenly notice mud, sand, water, or oil, you should straighten up as quickly as possible and ride around the spot while braking then lean back into the corner making sure you can still get around it. Cycling through a slippery spot while leaning usually causes the wheels to skid, particularly if you brake on the slippery patch while leaning.

Cornering in the rain

Conditions in the rain are completely different than on dry roads, with the result that corners must be taken a lot more carefully and slowly. When racing in the rain, cyclists slowly get to grips with the highest possible cornering speed during the first miles. Falls are most likely to occur when it starts raining during the race, as the high cornering speeds in the dry phase are dangerously high in the wet. All kinds of manhole covers and road markings become very dangerous in the rain, which have been the downfall of many riders, and not just in races. Wet corners in normally hot countries are very dangerous, as a greasy film of dust and motor oil can transform the roads into slides in wet weather. When racing in the rain, reduce the tire pressure slightly in order to increase the contact surface. You can read more about improving cornering technique in the technique training section.

8.7   Proper Shifting Technique

A long overdue technical advance during the 1980s made changing bicycle gears more simple. The correct shifting technique using modern gears is now limited to moving a lever or, in electronic models, to the simple touch of a button. However, the technology does not take away the need to decide when to change gear, which is still up to the cyclist. In order to avoid excessive wear and tear on the sprockets and sprocket wheel, when you change gears you should take the pressure off slightly (reduce pedal pressure). At low cadences, even modern gear systems work badly.

Gear ergonomics

A look at the ergonomics of the gear system only produces uniformity when braking, although the levers may be shaped differently. Small hands find it hard to cope with Shimano levers and would find Campagnolo and SRAM easier, or even the smaller ladies, STI levers by Shimano.

However, a rethink is called for when it comes to changing gear and when it comes to moving from one system to another. If you have learned on Campagnolo gears, it is initially harder to get used to Shimano, and those who are used to Shimano find SRAM difficult to use. This is also completely normal, and the automated movement patterns are only formed after about 700 miles or 500 gear shifts.

For racing cyclists, the issue of how many gears can be changed simultaneously in circuit races, attacks, and sprints is important. The three manufacturers differ considerably in this respect.

With Shimano, you can shift up by up to two gears but only one gear down per lever movement in sprints. SRAM manage two cogs when shifting up and only one shifting down, like Shimano. Campagnolo clearly wins out in practice and allows you to shift up by up to three gears and down by up to five gears with a single hard push of a button. However, this only applies to the top models.

How often do you change gear?

Shifters tempt you to change gear frequently, which is desirable in a race but not necessary in training. You should shift gears in the right situations and, above all, at the right time (e.g., before corners, blind sections, or a climb). It is not uncommon for cyclists to fall at unexpectedly steep climbs, because they are unable to change gears on the mountain with high pedal pressure and low cadence. In this case, you should turn around, change gears, and then resume cycling in the race direction. A diagonal chain line (i.e., large chainwheel in front and large sprocket behind) should be avoided as it increases friction loss and wear and tear.

The right gear ratio

The choice of the right gear ratio depends mainly on the situation, and also on cadence. The choice of gear ratio helps adapt your individual form to the terrain, situation, and wind conditions. In both racing and training (with the exception of certain types of training), the cadence should be around 90 rpm, and sometimes in training even higher. On the track, the racing cadence is significantly higher than in road racing, between 110 and 150 rpm depending on the discipline. The idea is therefore to choose a gear ratio depending on the speed, terrain, form, and training goal that allows you to keep to 90 rpm.

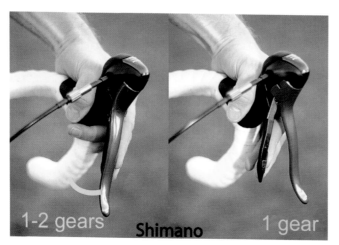

1-2 gears **Shimano** 1 gear

Shimano: In the STI lever by Shimano, you shift gears with the brake lever into a larger sprocket, with the smaller black index finger lever the chain moves down. On the left derailleur side the logic is the other way around.

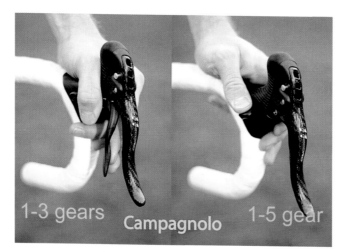

1-3 gears **Campagnolo** 1-5 gear

Campagnolo: The ErgoPower lever is operated by two gear levers. With the index finger behind the brake lever you shift into an easier gear ,and the thumb lever shifts into a harder gear. On the left derailleur side the logic is also reversed, the thumb switch moves the chain to a smaller chainwheel.

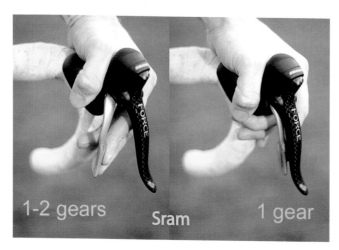

1-2 gears **Sram** 1 gear

SRAM: The double top lever has a dual function. Lightly touching with the index finger leads to a chain shift to a smaller sprocket. Harder pressure on the lever with longer lever path to a larger sprocket. On the left derailleur side, the logic is reversed.

High gears

However, there are cyclists who ride with extremely high gear ratios and low cadence; these riders usually have an unusually high power potential. A common error among newcomers to the sport and recreational cyclists is using excessively high gear ratios, meaning that they are basically training with the large wheel. This not only considerably reduces the training effect but also significantly increases the strain on the musculoskeletal system.

Gear meters

The following table shows the gear ratios commonly used in cycling with their corresponding meters of development. The distance traveled is shown for each complete crank rotation.

The development is calculated using the following simple formula: wheel circumference (C in meters) x ratio of front sprocket teeth divided by rear sprocket teeth.

Development = C x Sf / Sr

Example: 2.10 m x 53/15 = 7.42 m

When putting together your individual sprocket sizes, a gear ratio table is particularly useful in order to avoid overlaps between the large and small wheels. In race cycling circles, for flat races the close-ratio gears are favored (11-12-13-14-15-16-17-18-19-21), which enable very small increments of development. A gear ratio table is also necessary to determine the respective maximum permissible gear ratios in under-18 age groups. In order to be sure you are doing the right thing, use the rollout method (the distance a bike travels backward in a straight line through one full pedal revolution when the bicycle is in its largest gear). The wheel circumference should be measured accurately, as ultimately you will use this value when you calculate development.

Table 8.2: Gear meters of development table for a wheel circumference of 213.7 cm

Front ——→

Rear ——→

Rear \ Front	54	53	52	51	50	49	48	47	46	45	44	43	42	41	40	39	38	37	36
12	8.62	9.44	9.26	9.08	8.90	8.73	8.55	8.37	8.19	8.01	7.84	7.66	7.48	7.30	7.12	6.95	6.77	6.59	6.41
13	8.88	8.71	8.55	8.38	8.22	8.05	7.89	7.73	7.56	7.40	7.23	7.07	6.90	6.74	6.58	6.41	6.25	6.08	5.92
14	8.24	8.09	7.94	7.78	7.63	7.48	7.33	7.17	7.02	6.87	6.72	6.56	6.41	6.26	6.11	5.95	5.80	5.65	5.50
15	7.69	7.55	7.41	7.27	7.12	6.98	6.84	6.70	6.55	6.41	6.27	6.13	5.98	5.84	5.70	5.56	5.41	5.27	5.13
16	7.21	7.08	6.95	6.81	6.68	6.54	6.41	6.28	6.14	6.01	5.88	5.74	5.61	5.48	5.34	5.21	5.08	4.94	4.81
17	6.79	6.66	6.54	6.41	6.29	6.16	6.03	5.91	5.78	5.66	5.53	5.41	5.28	5.15	5.03	4.90	4.78	4.65	4.53
18	6.41	6.29	6.17	6.05	5.94	5.82	5.70	5.58	5.46	5.34	5.22	5.11	4.99	4.87	4.75	4.63	4.51	4.39	4.27
19	6.07	5.96	5.85	5.74	5.62	5.51	5.40	5.29	5.17	5.06	4.95	4.84	4.72	4.61	4.50	4.39	4.27	4.16	4.05
20	5.77	5.66	5.56	5.45	5.34	5.24	5.13	5.02	4.92	4.81	4.70	4.59	4.49	4.38	4.27	4.17	4.06	3.95	3.85
21	5.50	5.39	5.29	5.19	5.09	4.99	4.88	4.78	4.68	4.58	4.48	4.38	4.27	4.17	4.07	3.97	3.87	3.77	3.66
22	5.25	5.15	5.05	4.95	4.86	4.76	4.66	4.57	4.47	4.37	4.27	4.18	4.08	3.98	3.89	3.79	3.69	3.59	3.50
23	5.02	4.92	4.83	4.74	4.65	4.55	4.46	4.37	4.27	4.18	4.09	4.00	3.90	3.81	3.72	3.62	3.53	3.44	3.34
24	4.81	4.72	4.63	4.54	4.45	4.36	4.27	4.18	4.10	4.01	3.92	3.83	3.74	3.65	3.56	3.47	3.38	3.29	3.21
25	4.62	4.53	4.44	4.36	4.27	4.19	4.10	4.02	3.93	3.85	3.76	3.68	3.59	3.50	3.42	3.33	3.25	3.16	3.08
26	4.44	4.36	4.27	4.19	4.11	4.03	3.95	3.86	3.78	3.70	3.62	3.53	3.45	3.37	3.29	3.21	3.12	3.04	2.96
27	4.27	4.19	4.12	4.04	3.96	3.88	3.80	3.72	3.64	3.56	3.48	3.40	3.32	3.25	3.17	3.09	3.01	2.93	2.85
28	4.12	4.05	3.97	3.89	3.82	3.74	3.66	3.59	3.51	3.43	3.36	3.28	3.21	3.13	3.05	2.98	2.90	2.82	2.75
29	3.98	3.91	3.83	3.76	3.68	3.61	3.54	3.46	3.39	3.32	3.24	3.17	3.09	3.02	2.95	2.87	2.80	2.73	2.65
30	3.85	3.78	3.70	3.63	3.56	3.49	3.42	3.35	3.28	3.21	3.13	3.06	2.99	2.92	2.85	2.78	2.71	2.64	2.56
31	3.72	3.65	3.58	3.52	3.45	3.38	3.31	3.24	3.17	3.10	3.03	2.96	2.90	2.83	2.76	2.69	2.62	2.55	2.48
32	3.61	3.54	3.47	3.41	3.34	3.27	3.21	3.14	3.07	3.01	2.94	2.87	2.80	2.74	2.67	2.60	2.54	2.47	2.40

8.8   Overcoming Obstacles

When cycling on the roads, various different obstacles like potholes, drains, ties, stones, branches, or curbs can make it difficult to cycle safely. With a bit of practice, you can take these obstacles in stride by first putting the cranks in a horizontal position and gripping the handlebar either on the hoods or on the drops. The first movement is to get off the saddle and shift your bodyweight downward by bending your upper body forward and bending your elbows; then yank the handlebar and pedals as high as possible by raising your upper body, straightening your knees, and pulling your feet up by bending your knees, without trashing the handlebar. As you land, your body yields in order to absorb the shock.

Learning to jump

To learn this technique, first try lifting just the front or rear wheel off the ground. After more practice, combine both movements so that you jump. If you would like to jump over a high obstacle, you should ride really fast up to the obstacle (30 km/hr) so that you gain height and above all distance. High curbs should be negotiated slowly by pulling up the front wheel and then the rear wheel. Railroad tracks should be crossed as perpendicular as possible, but never at a sharp angle. If you need to cross tough terrain such as bumpy road surfaces, shift your bodyweight toward the rear wheel, extend your arms, and slide behind the saddle.

8.9   Technique Training With Young Cyclists

Cycling technique training with young cyclists and beginners should be prioritized within the overall training program. The younger (both in real age and in training age) the cyclist, the more cycle technique training should be carried out, so as to prepare for as many dangerous situations as possible in training and racing. Young cyclists find it relatively easy to learn technically demanding movements such as jumping, physical contact when cycling, or the standstill, due to their very favorable motor learning conditions (movement learning), and in fact the years between 10 and 14 are known as the golden learning age. The bike tourist or occasional cyclist should not shy away from trying one or more of these exercises for themselves as they will significantly improve their bike mastery and road safety.

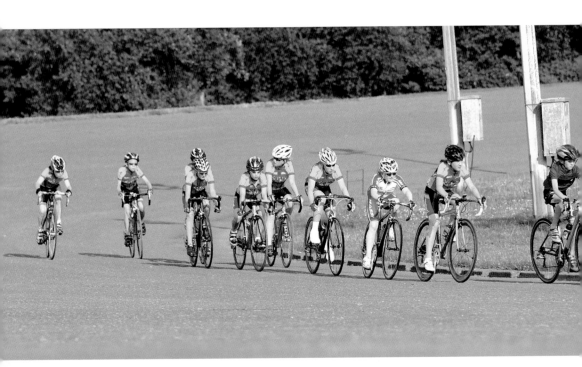

Technique training with kids

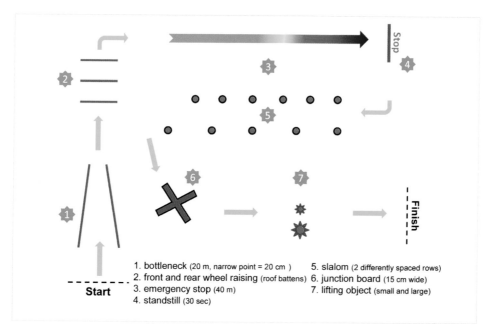

1. bottleneck (20 m, narrow point = 20 cm)
2. front and rear wheel raising (roof battens)
3. emergency stop (40 m)
4. standstill (30 sec)

5. slalom (2 differently spaced rows)
6. junction board (15 cm wide)
7. lifting object (small and large)

Fig. 8.15: Obstacle course

Obstacle course

Youth riders in particular find building an obstacle course very engaging and enjoyable despite incurring a few bruises in the process. Before practicing on the roads, find a firm grassy field on which falling is less painful. A tartan surface is also ideal. Allow your imagination free reign when designing the exercises; they should be practiced individually before performing them as a relay or timed one after the other. On the field, games like bike ball (with the feet) or catch can be attempted. In group training on a traffic-free road or a large empty car park, you can practice rear wheel touching, and the more advanced can try body touching (leaning on each other) while riding along as well as playing tag in teams of two. This includes riding with no hands, jumps, and standstills. All these exercises help to improve bike control, some specifically for a certain technique and others in general.

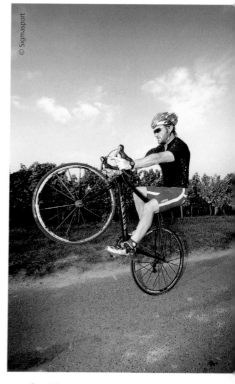

Perfect bike mastery

8.10 Road Safety in Traffic

How safely a cyclist moves in traffic depends mainly on his technical cycling skills. If you obey traffic rules, ride defensively and proactively, and control your bike, then with a very few exceptions, nothing will happen to you. In many critical situations, swerving is far preferable to a dangerous emergency stop followed by a possible crash.

Accident statistics

Traffic research has shown that most bicycle accidents are caused by cyclist's inattention or poor road conditions (e.g., potholes). Racing cyclists should always keep their eyes open and ride proactively with their wits about them, and they should interpret all hazardous traffic situations as potentially personally threatening, resulting in a defensive cycling style. It goes

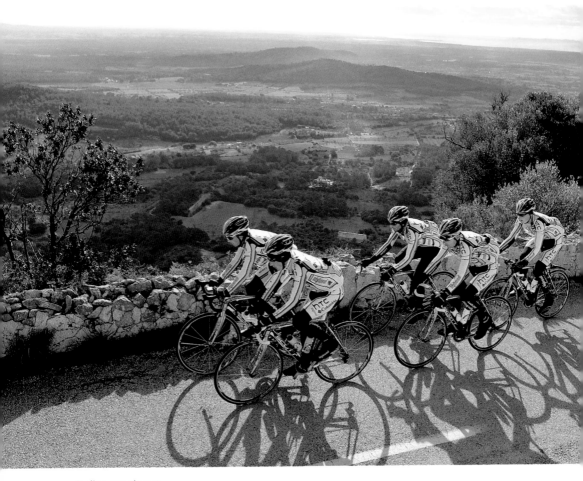

Cycling two abreast

without saying that you should wear a helmet, as there are no convincing arguments against this vital safety aid. However, it is also understandable that more senior cyclists who have ridden their bikes "topless" for many years with no problem find it hard to get used to wearing a helmet regularly. Young cyclists must of course wear a helmet not just when racing but also in training.

Cycling alone

If you cycle alone, always leave a safety margin of 1 to 3 feet to the side of the road to leave room for you to cycle around any hazards. As well as keeping an eye on oncoming traffic, you should also watch out for traffic coming from behind you by looking over your shoulder occasionally and by listening. If you are cycling down a road that is so narrow that a car overtaking a cyclist poses a danger to oncoming traffic, make yourself look wider than you really are

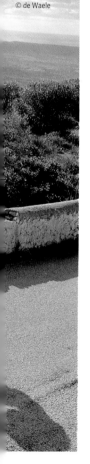

© de Waele

in order to prevent the car driver from thinking that they can overtake you quickly. This strategy can be a lifesaver, particularly in heavy city traffic.

Although according to road traffic regulations cycle paths must be used, it is up to the individual to judge whether he wants to expose himself to the additional danger of using a cycle path in city traffic.

At speeds of up to 20 km/hr, using a cycle path is no problem, but riding faster than this is risky. This is not due to the idea of cycle paths in itself, but the often ill-thought out implementation by planners. In the countryside, the use of cycle paths is usually not problematic.

Group training

Most rules for training alone also apply to group rides. It is important that the group stick together and do not take up a space more than100 yards long and 5 yards wide on the road. On very busy roads, it is advisable to ride in single file. On quieter roads, you can normally ride in a double paceline. This involves two cyclists riding side by side until they leave the leading position. The rider on the left falls behind and to the left after a few stronger pedal strokes (in order to pull away from the rider behind him), while the rider on the right does the same to the right. Once they have reached the back of the pack, they fall in line and cycle smoothly until they reach the front again. The leading cyclists should not try to pull away but keep up the same speed. Pulling away is the most common beginner's error in group training, leading to a loss of safety and smoothness.

Staggered cycling

In staggered cycling, you do not ride directly behind the rear wheel of the rider in front but always slightly offset behind him so that any pace fluctuations do not cause a crash. In addition, pace fluctuations can also be compensated for without braking. Do not look at the rear wheel of the rider in front of you, but look in front of you at shoulder height of the people in front and observe the traffic. If you would like, for example, to cycle out of the saddle you should do it very quickly and carefully to prevent the backward movement of your rear wheel endangering the cyclists behind you. Warning of obstacles can be given early on by the group (by calls or signals) and given a wide berth.

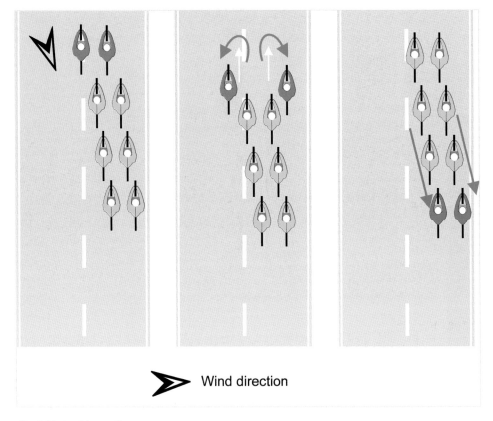

Wind direction

Fig. 8.16: Double paceline

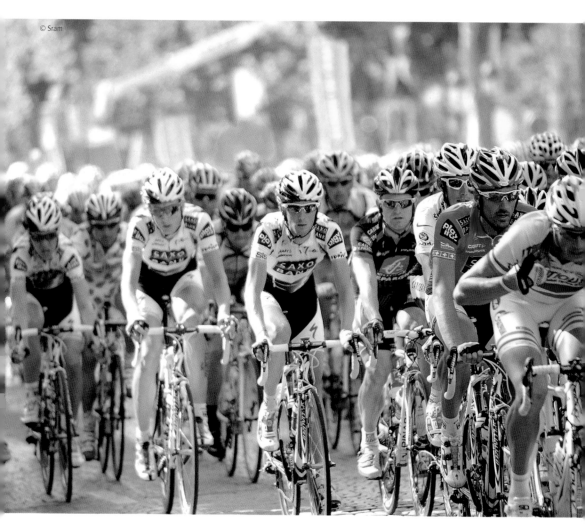

© Sram

In the race

In a race, try to stay in the first third of the pack in order to avoid the falls that usually take place in the middle or end of the pack. If you are not so sure of your cycling skills or those of your fellow cyclists, a position at the edge of the pack is recommended, where you have more room for maneuvering than jostling for position in the middle. You should keep far enough from the edge of the road or the curb so that you have enough room to maneuver in case of emergencies. Fast corners are usually safer on the inside rather than the outside, but avoid getting too close to the rear wheel of the rider in front but instead ride slightly offset back from him. In sticky situations, always keep a finger on the brakes. Surprising mass falls usually happen when nobody is expecting them, often when the pace is very slow and concentration levels drop to zero.

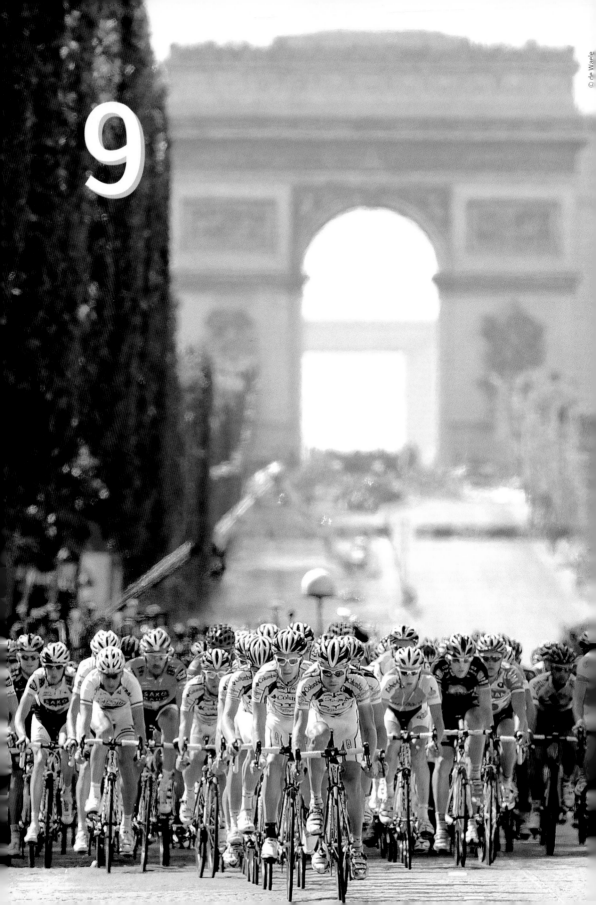

9

9   Tactics

9.1   Drafting and Echelons

Drafting

Drafting is an elementary cycling skill that must be mastered perfectly, as its labor-saving effect is the only way to enable high average speeds possible in long tours and races. The effort saved by drafting amounts to between 20% and 40%, and depends on many factors, such as speed, wind conditions, and the cyclist's weight.

Air resistance (drag) is proportional to the square of the speed, and this formula essentially means that drag increases more strongly than speed itself as the pace increases. For example, one cyclist who rides twice as fast as another cyclist experiences four times as much drag.

Saving 60%

An American study at the University of Florida found that the oxygen consumption and therefore the metabolic load of a cyclist in a slipstream at a speed of about 30 km/hr is about 18% lower than it would be if he were exposed to the wind. At a speed of 40 km/hr, the oxygen consumption is already around 27% lower than in the wind; in the pack in cycle races, for example, the intensity can even be about 39% less than at the front of the peloton. Behind a truck or tractor, this figure climbs to 60%. By clever use of slipstreaming, a huge amount of energy can therefore be saved; although this does not mean that you should shirk riding at the front of the peloton, as that would violate the code of honor that obliges the cyclist to do his share of the work at the front. However, it is the exception that proves the rule here.

Wheel sucker

In groups or in the peloton, it is possible to follow certain rules and ride cleverly to save energy without being called a wheel sucker. This is the term for a cyclist who rarely or never cycles at the front and then proceeds to go sprint past his fellow cyclists at the finish. This explains the sometimes surprising success of weaker cyclists who have a good sprint finish.

The aim of drafting is to ride as close as possible, but as safely as necessary, to the cyclist in front of you. At an even pace and when executed perfectly, as in team time trials, gaps of only a few inches are common. In groups in training or races, keep a lateral distance of 8 to 20 in.

The less stable you are, the greater the distance should be between you and the riders in front and beside you. The echelon bike formation stops you riding into the bike in front, improves visibility, and avoids the need to brake every time the pace changes, a little pressure on the pedals is sufficient.

Pulling off into the wind

The lead rider pulls off into the wind, which in still conditions or little wind often leads to confusion over which side to pull out. If there is little wind, the optimal drag must first be sought, and until a group has learned to work together, the distance should be slightly greater for safety reasons. Clear hand signs and communication are very useful here. Particularly in the case of beginners, it makes sense to be cautious because they are not familiar with pulling off and suddenly veering off, which can cause the whole paceline to pile up.

Echelon

The echelon is a phenomenon feared by both touring and racing cyclists, which always occurs when strong winds blow diagonally forward or sideways into a closed paceline or pack.

The echelon always lies on the downwind side of the road. Some riders then find a slipstream on one side of the road or on the whole width of the road in races, by spreading out against

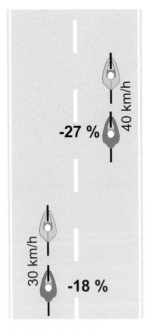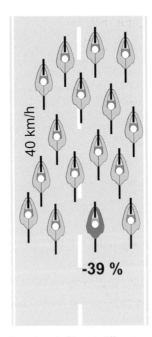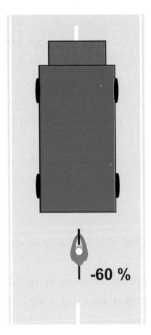

Fig. 9.1: Reduction in oxygen consumption when drafting at different speeds

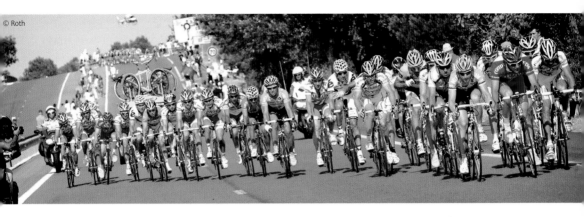

© Roth

the wind and rotating, while the other riders line up behind in an echelon like pearls on a necklace. For these riders, the slipstream of the leader is only minimal, so the echelon is very taxing for them. It often takes its toll on them, and gaps can appear.

Echelon victim

To avoid being an echelon victim, it is therefore important to ride near the front of the paceline, as the riders in the middle or at the back of the peloton usually have no chance of catching up with the leading paceline without their own. The only way of keeping in touch with the lead is by opening up one or more other pacelines as soon as possible, which then ride behind the leading echelon. It is often difficult to bring order to these groups in the form of a Belgian tourniquet as many cyclists are already riding at their limit and are unable to undertake any more leading work. The danger of falling in an echelon is greatly increased by cyclists who are struggling at their limit and is another reason never to ride at the back of a peloton in the wind.

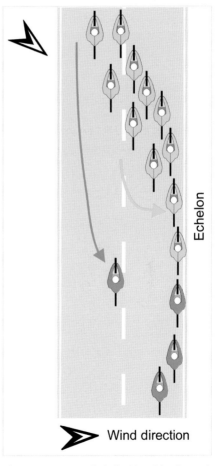

Fig. 9.2: In a crosswind, the blue riders have almost no slipstream and sooner or later will drop off the pace.

Rotating pacelines

Rotating pacelines in echelons are particularly common in the windy spring classics in which the sometimes huge starting fields are so severely decimated by the wind that it is not uncommon for only a few riders to reach the finish.

In smaller groups, a formation in which the group lines up against the wind and the riders regularly rotate has proven to be successful. Cycling diagonally behind the rider in front, you ride in their slipstream to gain some respite from the hard work of leading. The higher the tempo and the more riders in the group, the shorter the time spent in the lead. There is no real difference between this and the Belgian tourniquet.

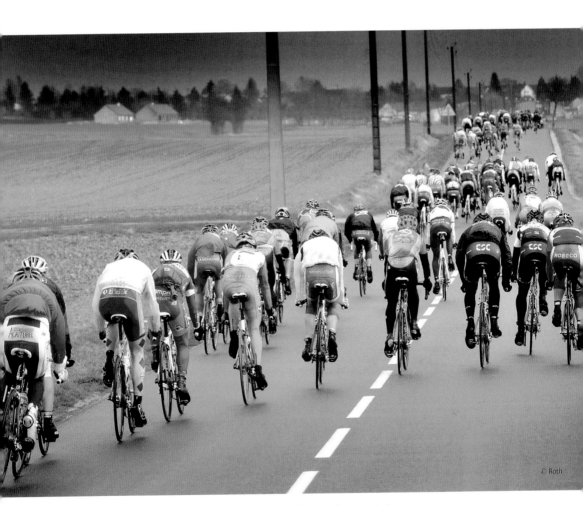

© Roth

It is common for small groups, called rotating pacelines, to form in windy races.

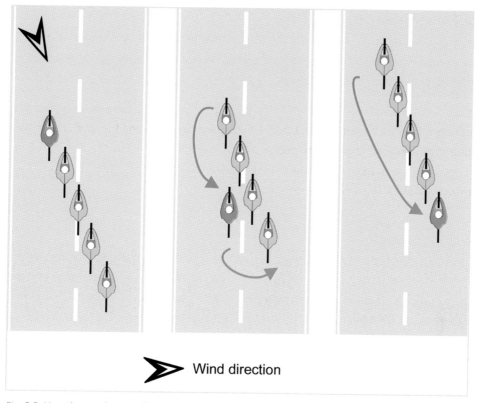

Fig. 9.3: How the rotating paceline works

Regular rotation

The first rotation description is for a group of three to six cyclists: If there is a crosswind, the cyclists ride staggered diagonally behind each other so that their shoulder is level with the hip of the rider in front. The more head-on the wind, the less the riders' bikes overlap and the line stretches out. The cyclist taking over the lead maintains the previous pace until he is replaced by the rider behind.

When pulling off, you leave the front to the side the wind is coming from and, reducing your speed very slightly but without losing too much pace, fall back to the end of the group; then increase your pedal pressure briefly as you join it on the side protected from the wind. The time spent at the front can vary from 30 seconds to several minutes. To avoid splitting up the group, stronger cyclists do not ride faster but lead for longer than weaker riders. For a group to function effectively, an even pace is essential, as it only takes one rider to fall behind or be unwilling or unable to take the lead and deliberately or due to his incapacity spoils the group and prevents harmonious collaboration and the success of the group.

Everything for the group

In races, riders must first subordinate their own interests and place their strength entirely at the service of the group. Even in bike touring, a group that works well together makes a training ride or tour much more enjoyable.

Riders who are unwilling or unable to should not lead but should leave a gap for the rider pulling off from the front to the back. The rotating paceline or Belgian tourniquet is used in all team time trial races.

The technique of the **double paceline** has already been described in chapter 8.10. The double paceline is the recommended organizational structure for large training groups.

Belgian tourniquet

The Belgian tourniquet is practically the same as the rotating paceline and is so-called as this formation is particularly common in the spring classics in often poor weather conditions in the cycling nation of Belgium. In the Belgian tourniquet, a large group of riders who either find themselves in a breakaway attempt or as the victims of an echelon are trying to either catch up with the rest of the group or the lead as quickly as possible. Particularly in the lower categories, many riders find it hard to master the group technique of rotating, thereby incurring the wrath of their teammates.

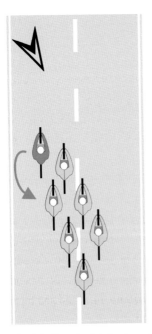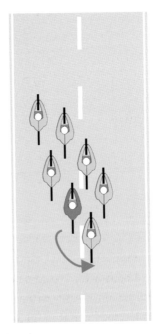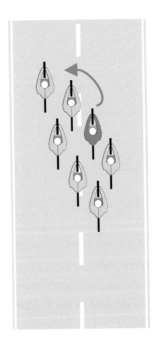

Fig. 9.4: How the Belgian tourniquet works

Rotating paceline

A rotating paceline must consist of at least five riders if it is to work well. The rotating paceline is characterized by a fast to very fast pace. Leading consists only of a brief spell in front so that every rider is only exposed to the wind for only a short time. It consists of two lines riding side by side at different speeds: The line facing the wind falls back at a slightly slower speed thereby providing a slipstream for the faster line.

When taking over the lead, you ride past the rider in front of you who is about to pull off and peel off downwind from the faster line; carry on pedaling at a slightly lower speed so that you now fall back into the other line and then finally join the end of the faster line. It is crucial when falling to the back to seek out the slipstream of the rider in front of you who is also falling to the back; the art of a smoothly functioning rotating paceline is to keep small gaps of equal size between the rider in front of you and the other line, as large gaps and pace fluctuations disturb the rhythm of the paceline.

Practicing the tourniquet

The riders create an elliptical path on their way through the Belgian tourniquet and, depending on the strength and direction of the wind, the paceline is spread over the entire width of the road. The idea is to practice the formation of the rotating paceline or echelon in training until it is perfect. The group must quickly reform and get into position according to the wind direction, particularly after corners.

For a rotating paceline to work correctly, it must be composed of experienced riders who have mastered the rotation technique. In races, it is common to see inexperienced riders who, due to their inability to form a well-functioning paceline or echelon, are unable to catch up with the relatively slow-moving peloton. Even breakaway groups with very good endurance fitness levels may not necessarily be able to form a good paceline for many different reasons, such as poor tactical skills, personal and team interests, or fitness problems. There are a few features of the rotating paceline that can occur during the course of a race.

The door opener

A door opener is the rider who cycles in the slipstream at the end of the echelon or paceline who opens the door for the cyclist falling back from the lead. In other words, the door opener allows him to reenter the paceline. The door opener's tasks consist of protecting and safeguarding the paceline in front of him. If nobody took responsibility for this, riders cycling behind the paceline trying to enter the echelon would easily be able to penetrate the group and force other cyclists out, disturbing the harmonious interaction of the group.

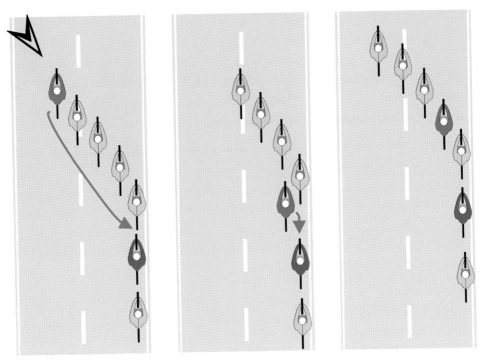

Fig. 9.5: The door opener allows the rider falling back from the lead to reenter the paceline.

A teammate should be selected for the role of door opener or a rider who is accepted by the group. However, the role is often taken on by a rider who does not wish to lead.

Upwind out of the lead

If no door opener is present and reentry into the paceline is repeatedly prevented by blocking riders, a different technique can be used: Do not pull away from the lead downwind but first accelerate upwind and then let yourself fall back in the slipstream of the paceline. Once you reach the echelon at the roadside, allow yourself to fall back carefully, and you will be sure of your place in the paceline, as the cyclists riding in the slipstream cannot defend themselves against a cyclist approaching from the front and must make room for him.

Now there are not only the situations in which you yourself ride in a paceline, but also those in which you are struggling against a crosswind and would like to have a place in the paceline. There are only two possibilities here: You either start a new paceline or try to join an existing one by taking advantage of the riders' loss of attention. Physical, bike, or handlebar contact is usually the cause of falls on echelons at the end of pacelines on these occasions.

Shaking off wheelsuckers

In most groups, there are a few riders who after a certain time are unwilling or unable to take the lead. Many attempts are then made to shake off these riders cycling at the end of the group by taking them in the echelon and raising the tempo slightly, which either shakes them off or reminds them to cooperate. Either way, these riders are forced into the lead by those riders next to them, allowing the gap to the group to increase. At some point, either you or the wheelsucker must close this gap. If several riders in the group are taking part in this maneuver, at some point it will be hard for the wheelsucker to close the gaps. Either he now cooperates or loses touch.

Disturbing the group

If you are in the situation where a teammate is at the front, the group's teamwork can be disturbed by gradually reducing the pace in the lead, pulling off incorrectly, drafting while leading, or allowing gaps to appear. Very soon, though, the other riders will notice and no longer allow the troublemaker to join their paceline.

9.2   Before the Race

In the week before a race, try to familiarize yourself with the course, if possible, so that you can memorize the most important sections. Windy sections (crosswinds), where it will probably be necessary to form echelons, or good places to attack can be identified and be considered when planning your racing tactics. If it is not possible to visit the course, at the very least you should familiarize yourself with the course profile using a map. Google maps aerial views or hybrid views provide accurate images of a race course. This not only applies to road races but also and particularly to circuit races.

Shortly before the race, or, if possible, beforehand on the event organizer's website, you can get an idea of the start list and memorize the numbers of the strong riders who you may be able to follow for tactical purposes. After a thorough warm-up (30-40 min), which is longer the shorter the race, and the other preparations (mental preparation, stretching, leg rubs, checking food supplies), proceed calmly to the start, where you should try to get as near to the front as possible, which in lower category races often means taking your place as much as 15 minutes before the start. The waiting time before the start can then be filled with a few stretching exercises.

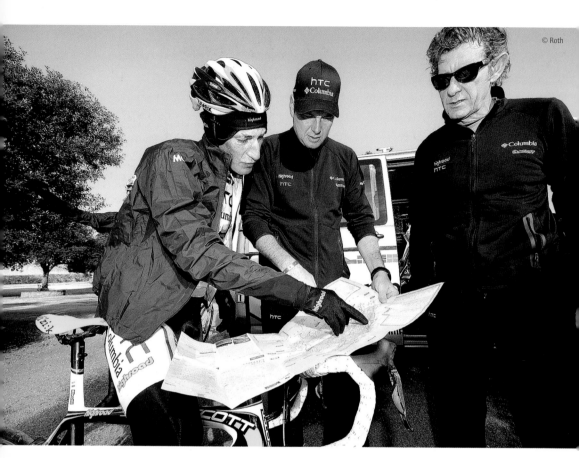

© Roth

Fig. 9.6: Checking the course prevents surprises.

9.3 During the Race

Races on short courses are characterized by fast starts, which can be the downfall of many a rider. If you have not warmed up thoroughly, you have no chance. Long road races usually have a fairly sedate starting tempo, during which you can prepare yourself for the hard work to follow with high pedal cadences. The different tactical situations that may occur during a race are described in detail in the following sections, and the explanations should help the less tactically experienced rider to find the right tactics. However, it should also be noted that a knowledge of tactical refinements and tricks does not necessarily mean that one is able to put them into practice. Usually a cyclist must first make every tactical error once in order to then react better the next time the situation arises. Here another factor comes into play along with tactical talent or quite simply a sense for the right situation, which is very hard to teach. In breakaway groups, particularly in youth categories or in the lower adult categories, there is often a significant tactical divide between seasoned, experienced, and completely green beginners. Often, good tactics enable the older more experienced riders to beat their younger rivals.

9.4   In the Pack

All the action is at the front of the pack and in the breakaway groups. You should therefore try to remain in the first third of the pack where you can actively participate in the race. In the rear third, the changes of pace are more pronounced (braking, accelerating after cornering) and the danger of falling for inattentive, tired riders is higher, and the possibility of becoming detached from the pack or entering the echelon is many times higher.

The position in the first third of the pack is linked with frequent changes of position particularly in the transition in the center of the pack. Riders push sideways into the front part of the pack and stream back into the center. When viewed from a great height, these movements in the peloton look very impressive. Basically, inexperienced riders feel safer at the edge of the pack than in the center.

In mountainous terrain, the leader determines the pace and stretches out the pack; the first to reach the top of the pass can make the descent calmly and with concentration, while the tail-enders often have to risk everything in order to catch up with the rest of the pack. Poor climbers try to get as near to the front as possible before the mountains so that they may even be able to set the pace, at least then you can allow yourself to fall back on the mountain and yet still reach the summit with the peloton.

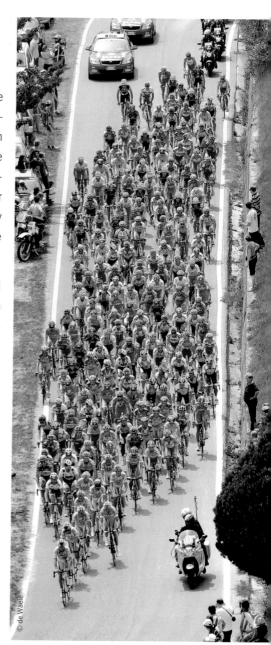

Apparent chaos, but without order and clear rules there would be many more falls.

If you have the possibility of climbing a mountain at the front of the field or a group, this has a very positive psychological effect, and you can set your own pace and you feel stronger. Climbs are tactically very important sections of road races, as breakaway groups or individual riders are often caught on climbs. Attacks, no matter how short, are usually carried out on climbs, because drafting is less important here than on the flat.

9.5   Breakaway Groups or Individual Attacks

While in U16 age-group races it is rare for breakaway groups to reach the finish and the winner is often decided after a mass sprint finish, group breakaways or individual attacks are more common in junior races, particularly in amateur and women's races. Young riders should be taught that the holy grail of cycling is a successful breakaway attempt and not a sprint at the end of a race which does not always result in victory.

Attacks

Attacks or breakaways are attempts to pull away from your competitors (peloton or group), be it to win a prime, catch up with a group, or just to place or win the race. There are many different reasons why riders attack. However, a lot of attacks are carried out in the wrong place or at the wrong time so that they are basically just a waste of energy. This absolutely does not mean that only the last, decisive attack is worthwhile, though, for many other previous attacks during the race may have contributed to the victory. Ultimately the saying holds true that nothing ventured, nothing gained. Breakaways in adverse situations just to impress coaches, team doctors, or parents are pointless and waste valuable energy.

When should attacks be used?

There is no one definitive answer to this question as there are a whole series of times at which attacks can be successful. The most conducive to success are the following:

- After an unsuccessful breakaway attempt, as soon as the riders are settled again
- Among slow, inattentive riders in the field
- If you are feeling very strong
- If your rivals are tired or not concentrating
- At or after fast pace

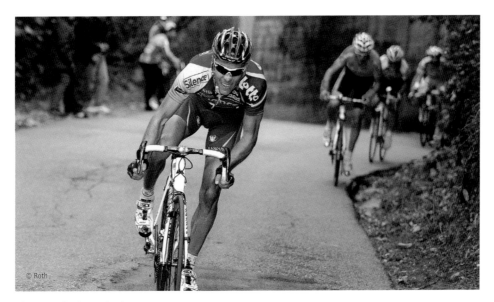

Most attacks do not lead to success.

However, an old rule states that you should only attack when you are suffering and in pain, as this is when your rivals are also struggling, and they may be unable or unwilling to react to your attack. During the course of a race it is normal to attack many times, of which only one will lead to victory.

Where is the right place for an attack?

The choice of place depends on what kind of rider you are: A climber will always attack on a steep incline, while a good descender attacks on a descent or the last yards of a climb, and a good individual time trialer on the flat. It is important to have good performance prerequisites for these specific situations (good climber), and as mentioned, wait for the right moment. Tactically advantageous points are just before corners, after a corner, into a headwind or crosswind, in technically difficult sections (corners, poor road surface), in the mountain, or in descents. Attacks following falls, equipment defects, or at food checkpoints are considered to be unsporting and are therefore obviously not advisable.

- Climb
- Top of the pass, summit, or descent
- After or before corners
- Echelon
- Winding sections

How do you attack?

Attacks should take your rivals by surprise. It would therefore not be smart to attack from the lead of the pack or a group, as then the element of surprise would be nonexistent. Only if a rider is very strong, and even then only in the mountains, can he attack from the front. However, it is possible to edge away from the front and then attack when there is a gap of a few yards between you and the other riders.

In a breakaway group, the best place to attack from is the back, and in a pack, attacks take place from the edge somewhere in the first third. In a group, let yourself fall back slightly, choose a suitable gear, attack and pull as fast as possible sideways out of the echelon so that you provide as little slipstream as possible to those chasing you. The surprise effect and high speed will quickly allow a gap of 20 to 50 yards that you must now build on. The attack itself must be explosive and flat out; the first 500 to 1,000 yards are covered at very high speeds and very high gear ratios. Only after that can you look around you and decide whether to carry on or let the others catch you. The first part of a breakaway is characterized by a very high heart rate and high oxygen consumption; part of the energy is provided anaerobically, leading to increased lactic acid production and muscle hyperacidity, so you should not ride too fast now to avoid too much energy being supplied anaerobically, which would prevent you from continuing the race. It is therefore essential to experiment with this situation in training in order to know how long and how fast you can ride with which feeling and even better with this heart rate in order to prevent a possible overloading (hyperacidity) that forces you to drop out.

Solo breakaways

Crossing the finishing line in the lead after a solo breakaway (short or long) is certainly the best feeling a cyclist can have, but it is also one of the hardest to achieve. The effort involved is similar to a time trial and should be as even as possible. Cycle with high cadences and high gear ratios at 85% to 90% of MHR in as aerodynamic a position as possible toward the finish or prime.

From a tactical point of view, there is really very little to bear in mind here. The only important thing is the careful organization of your energy so that you are caught just before the finish line. Poor sprinters in particular try just before the end of the race to reach the finish alone. Deciding factors here are also a perfect cornering technique and tires that grip well.

The breakaway group

In a breakaway group, at least two riders work more or less on reaching the finish together. More or less means that often not all the riders in the group work together and only ride in the group's paceline for team tactical or personal reasons.

The previously mentioned drafting techniques are used here. The effect on the group is positive if experienced riders take over the organization of the group and get the echelon or paceline going using concise commands. It is common for completely different intentions and performance levels to come up against each other in breakaway groups, and these groups are usually doomed to fail. If a group breaks away and you are not sure whether to join them, first consider the composition of the group. Does it include all the important teams and their strongest riders? Is the successful rider xy with the instinct for choosing the right group part of it? If the answer to these questions is yes, you should try to join the group. However, many groups are just used by the stronger teams to keep the pace fast and have no hope of a chance.

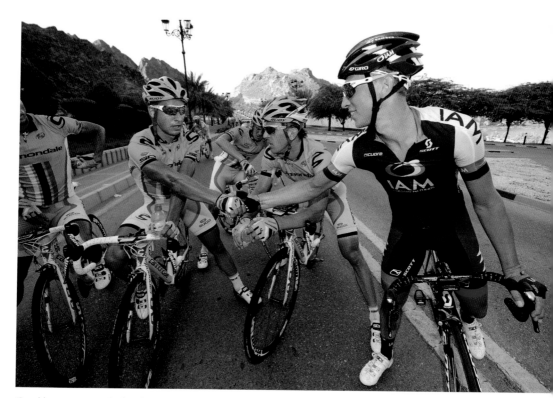

Good losers congratulating the winner

9.6   The Finish

The finish nearly always involves a sprint, with the only exception being when a solo break-away rider finishes ahead of the others. Even when only two riders are sprinting for victory or to place, there are a lot of tactical nuances to bear in mind, without which you can only win if you are the physically superior rider. The situation in a mass sprint is more difficult, and this is explored in more detail next.

In a sprint, the decisions concerning tactical behavior must be made so quickly that there is no time to weigh all the different strategies. It is usually impossible to correct tactical decisions once they have been made. So, it is important to wait for the right time at the start of your own tactical moves, as the only other option is to react to your rivals' tactics.

Only the experienced cyclist can draw on a variety of tactical moves that enable him to beat his opponent despite being in worse shape. This is why tactical training is very important for beginners in order to reduce the experienced cyclists' advantage in this area.

Types of sprinter

There are two main types of sprinter: the final velocity sprinter who needs a relatively long distance (550 yd) to reach full speed but who can maintain it for a very long time, and the explosive sprinter who can develop his highest speeds over a short distance (110-220 yd). Such riders may, for example, enter a final corner in fifth place and win the race with a final spurt, however short. There is a whole range of intermediate types between these two extremes.

Riders who are sure that they could never sprint usually belong to the category that needs a long distance to reach full speed. Furthermore, the individual highest speed of these riders is lower than that of good sprinters. Better sprinting is achieved by increased speed, speed strength, and strength endurance training and also improved tactical behavior.

Sprinting in pairs

If two riders have a sufficiently large lead, a tactical battle in which both cyclists ride very slowly keeping an eye each other begins. The slow sprinter used to tours will try to keep the pace as fast as possible and start his sprint as soon as possible, while the explosive sprinter will wait as long as possible then catch the other rider in the final yards of the race. In general, the rear position is preferable as it allows you to react better to your rival's actions and also to benefit from his slipstream. Try to reach your opponent's rear wheel so that you can implement your own tactics and not depend on his.

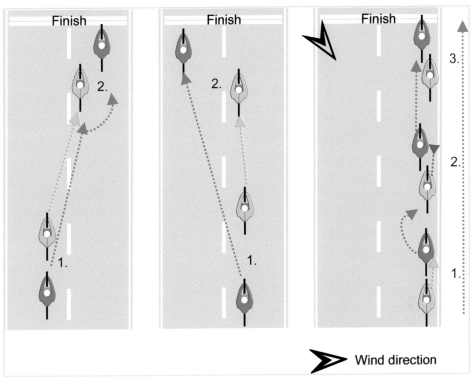

Fig. 9.7: Sprint in a pair. 1. The rear rider remains in the slipstream and then pulls past. 2. The rear rider allows a gap to form, then attacks suddenly and overtakes the leader at high speed so that the latter is unable to follow him. 3. The door opener in a sprint.

Windy conditions produce a very interesting tactical variation. In this case, both riders ride in a crosswind, and the rear one must ride upwind in order to pass the leader.

If you start the sprint from the rear position from the middle of the road, ride quickly into the crosswind so as to allow the rear rider as little slipstream as possible. Even if you start your sprint from the front, you must still ride into the crosswind at the side of the road.

Door open and shut

If the sprint is in full swing, the front rider can offer the back one an apparent possibility of passing him in his slipstream. To this end, the leader opens the door by pulling off slightly toward the middle of the road, just far enough to give the rear rider the impression that he can pass him.

When the rear rider now tries to push into the gap, the front rider closes the door again by pulling back to the side of the road or curb and forces the other riders to take the pressure off the pedals slightly but without endangering the rider behind him. This quick maneuver is usually enough to retain the lead right up to the finish, as the other rider must now try again to pull ahead into the wind, but the finish is now usually too close for this.

Group sprint (three or more cyclists)

Most of the aforementioned tactics also apply to sprints in larger groups. It is usually already apparent from intermediate spurts or attacks who the strongest sprinter of the group is. If possible, as a weaker sprinter you should stick to his back wheel over the final miles for as long as possible and attack when he attacks. Although you may have no chance of overtaking him, you can still try to stay in his slipstream and finish in a good position. Speed demons usual-ly still try to break away in the final miles, which is sometimes successful due to a lack of atten-tion on the part of the other riders. The attack should begin undetected at the end of the group in order to surprise the others and not be launched too soon.

The element of surprise

If the sprint has not already begun (600-200 yd before the finish), a weaker sprinter can use this surprise tactic to open up such a wide gap between himself and the group that he can re-tain his lead right to the finish. If this does not work for the weaker sprinter, he should join the front of the paceline and try to sprint from the front of the group, which usually allows him to achieve a better result than if he were to start his sprint from the back of the group.

In a sprint from the middle of the group, you should take care not to be boxed in so that you are unable to use your sprinting strength. The ideal positions for the sprint are second to fourth where you can only rarely be boxed in. In any case, it is better to decide on a tactic and imple-ment it with all your strength (e.g., attacks from the end of the group) rather than just doing it half-heartedly. This requires courage, putting yourself on the line, and possibly crossing the finish line last in your group. The absolute determination to implement your chosen tactics with all your power usually mobilizes your last reserves and contributes to success (chapter 7). He who hesitates is lost!

Mass sprint

The sight of a tight group sprinting is impressive and unpredictable, and falls are not uncommon. The danger of being boxed in or blocked is significant in a mass sprint, which is why during the final miles it is essential to be at the front of the pack (second row), as this is the only place from which you can react to sudden attacks and advances and look for the right rear wheel to

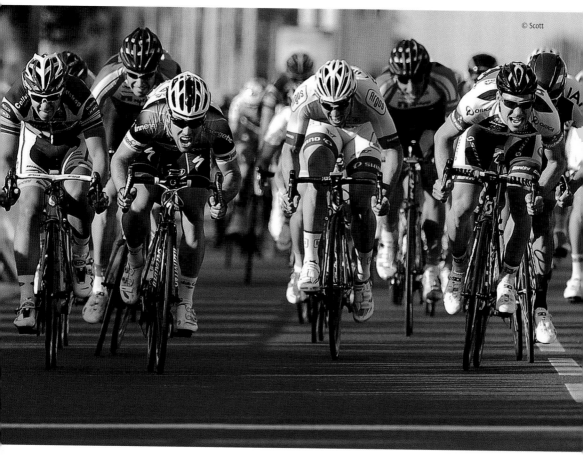

© Scott

Mass sprint

ride behind in the final spurt. The same rules apply here as for the two-man sprint (door open–door shut; crosswind). Sprinters with a strong team behind them are clearly at an advantage. As it is the role of the team to prepare and move its sprinter forward for the final spurt, it is almost impossible to penetrate the phalanx of this group. If you are riding on your own, you should cycle as near as possible to the rear wheel of a sprinter in a good position.

All sprinters to the front!

In the event of a mass sprint, all the sprinters gather at the front of the peloton in the final miles. Herein lies the chance of an outsider who is not a strong sprinter to overthrow the sprinters' plans with a well-timed attack. If no team makes the pace for its sprinters, the pace is not usually fast enough to make a breakaway impossible. The gathered sprinters then keep each other in check with counterattacks so as not to waste their chance for the sprint.

A teammate who pulls you to a sprint in an echelon, opens the door, and then shuts it is in any case very useful. In all sprints, particular in the peloton, you must stick to the riding line to avoid endangering other riders. Weaving all over the road is as unsporting as it is dangerous. Cyclists often make the mistake of stopping pedaling a few yards before the finish line, which can easily cost them the victory or place they thought was theirs.

Tiger pounce

In mass sprints directly before the finish, several riders may be level with each other so that a tiger pounce is required for victory. This involves pushing the bike forward explosively by extending the arms and legs and simultaneously sliding off the back of the saddle. In cycling, the winner is the one whose front edge of the front wheel is perpendicular to the finish line. The tiger pounce is all about timing, as if it is executed too early or too late, you give away valuable inches and thereby the victory, so it should also be practiced in training.

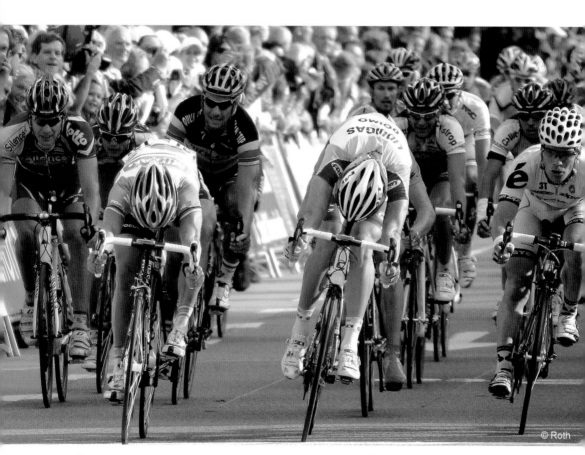

Tiger pounce

9.7   Team Tactics

Cycling is not only a classic individual sport but is often ridden as a team tactical race, particularly at professional level, to the extent that it is now almost impossible to win a race without the help of a team. The top individual riders need the support of their teammates when sprinting, in breakaways, or in the mountains in order to eventually win out. Even amateur and women's races feature strengthened teams not only in national leagues but also in the lower and even youth categories. The negative aspect of these often very strong teams is that they are able to completely dictate the race in small races and win most of the primes and prize money, so races become boring. Smaller teams or individual riders therefore have little chance of finishing on the podium.

Team talk

The team should develop appropriate race tactics before the start, which may be deviated from if necessary. It is often a bad idea to choose a rider in advance who all the other riders work for, as this rider may then go on to perform badly. It is better to take the decision on which rider to support during the race.

If one or two riders in a team find themselves in a leading group, the task of their teammates riding in the peloton consists either of slowing down the peloton by cutting back the pace slightly at the front (before corners) or trying to thwart any attacks, which is usually more effective. This involves immediately following the attacking riders and, after reaching their rear wheel, undertaking no more leading work until the group or solo rider has closed the gap to the leading group or until they have been pulled back into the group again. This team tactic is used until the breakaway group with teammates has built up an unassailable lead. However, if you are able to draw level with the leading group with your colleagues at the rear wheel of a rival, you are now in a position to attack. It is important that during the breakaway of a teammate nobody else from his team attacks at the same time.

Sprint preparation

In order to create the best possible prerequisites for a sprint, in the last miles before an intermediate sprint or before the finish the team rides so fast that an attack is impossible. This involves several riders riding flat out in a line. Tired riders gradually drop back until only the last teammates and the sprinter remain. In the final yards, the door method is used, making it more difficult for the other riders to catch the lead sprinter. If you are part of a two-man or even three-man breakaway, as far as possible take it in turns to attack over the final miles until one rider from the team is finally able to pull ahead.

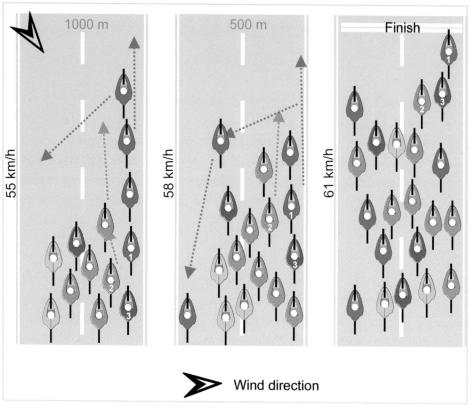

Fig. 9.8: Perfect team preparation for a sprint. Just before the finish, the sprinter's rivals are forced to cover a greater distance.

9.8 Tactical Situations in Different Types of Races

Criteriums

Entries for criteriums, or crits, are usually lower than for road races. In the European format, points can be scored after certain laps during the race, with 5, 3, 2, and 1 point and double points for the end sprint. Due to the frequent awarding of points and the primes given for winning intermediate laps, the speed in criteriums is very high. In order to retain an overview of these often-confusing races, you should ride near the front.

In small pelotons it is possible to rest for a few laps in the center or at the end of the pack, as you can regain the lead within the space of a lap. The tactically inexperienced can get their bearings from the sprinters or criterium specialists. Poor sprinters attack quite reasonably after a prime or a points lap in order to ride for a few laps at the front of the field and win a point, as they have no chance of winning points in the very hotly contested sprints.

From a team tactical point of view, criteriums are one of most difficult types of race. Only with a good overview, ideally with the help of a coach who is making notes, is it possible to have several riders placing well up the field. The coach gives tactical instructions to this end, as he is the only person who knows the exact point total of all the riders. It is not uncommon for coaches and riders to communicate via secret signs or boards with coded instructions.

Circuit races

The tactical situation in circuit races, particularly with short laps, is similar to that in criteriums. Race-deciding breakaways may rarely take place right at the start of the race, but usually the race is decided near the middle or even in the final laps.

For a group to work well, the number of riders is important, as it has been demonstrated time and again that groups that are too big (from about 8-10 riders) only rarely have a chance of finishing, due to the conflicting interests of the riders. In large groups, the number of riders who never lead increases; they can hide away at the end of the group, thus preventing harmonious collaboration. Groups of three to six riders are considered to be ideal. Attacks shortly after high primes have often proved successful.

Road races

Road races usually feature large to very large fields, which is why at tactically advantageous points (echelon, climbs) it is better to be at the front so that you don't get left behind when the field separates. The peloton is often split into several groups, and even larger groups have a chance here. High-level road races are largely influenced by the team tactics of the strongest teams. The information given above on echelons or rolling pacelines is particularly relevant for road races.

Individual time trials

In individual time trials, there are very few tactical rules to bear in mind. The most important of these is to spread your energy correctly so that you don't run out of steam prematurely. High cadences (85-100 rpm) are ridden with very high gear ratios; there is little gear changing so that the rhythm is not interrupted. Any wind protection (walls, hedges, trees) should be used; corners should be ridden on the ideal line.

Time-trial training is very important for a good time trial performance, as only when you know your individual endurance performance limit are you able to accurately determine the speed you can ride at in a race without jeopardizing or ruining your performance. Mental race preparation is very important in time trials (see chapter 7). The aim is to start the race in a performance-affirming, positive, slightly aggressive but still relaxed frame of mind. Even during the race, the rider must remain both mentally and physically relaxed.

Team time trials

Most of the specific characteristics of time trials have already been mentioned in the previous section. For team time trials, however, there are additional tactical aspects to be considered. For example, the team should as much as possible be composed of equally strong riders, who also have similar physiques. If there are big differences, a shorter rider should always ride behind a taller one, unless the shorter rider is stronger than the rest of the group. Rotation (see paceline) must be practiced to perfection in training, and the riders' sequence should be the same in training and competition.

The riders only lead for 20 to 30 seconds and then drop back to the end of the paceline. When you come into the lead, you should never increase the pace as otherwise the rider who has just dropped back will have trouble joining the end of the paceline. Critical for success is an even pace, as pace fluctuations would exhaust the weakest team members and may force them to drop out. Although a good result can still be achieved even with three riders, the aim should be for the whole team to reach the finish line. A team must experiment in training to determine its maximal sustainable speed in order to be able to ride at exactly this speed during a race.

© Scott

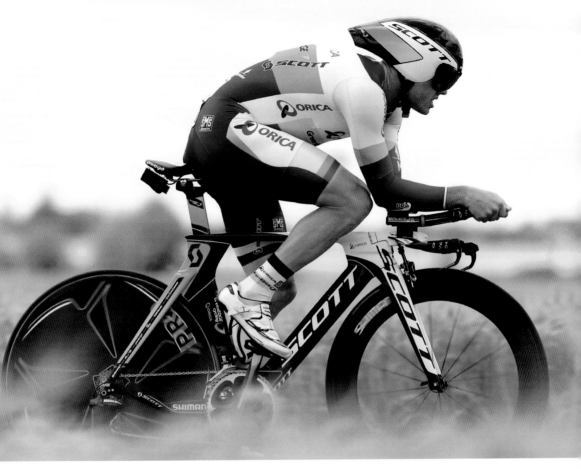

Time trials

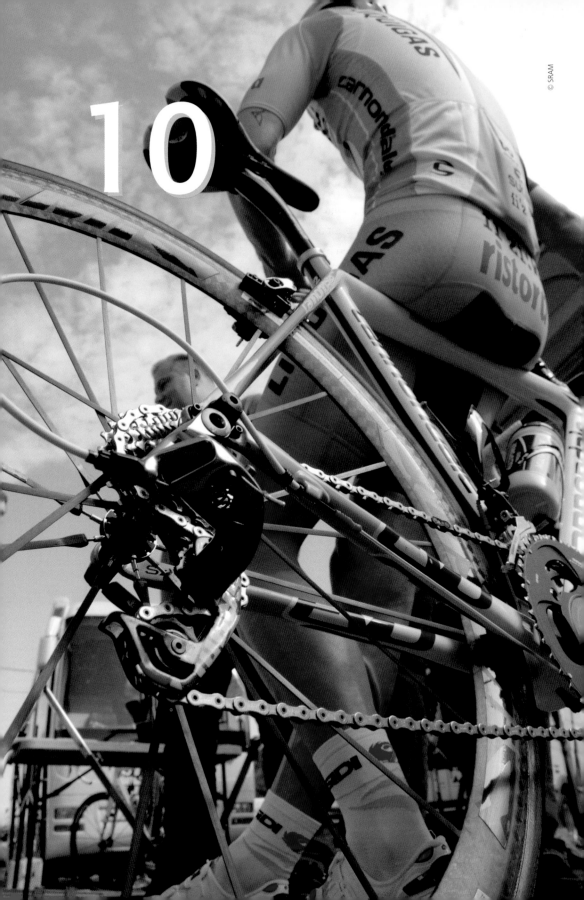

10

© SRAM

10   Equipment

10.1   Racing Bike and Frame

The huge choice of manufacturers and models, added to a lack of expert knowledge, makes purchasing a racing bike very daunting for a newcomer to the sport. It is often hard for a lay-person to understand what a salesperson is saying, so the basic terms and ideas are explained here. This basic knowledge of bike technology will make your search much easier. However, current equipment tests and ratings are not included. For this you should consult a monthly cycling magazine that publishes very detailed test results.

Frame and fork

The frame is the heart of the bike and distributes the rider's weight over both wheels, and its design features allow the transmission of power from rider to bike while still retaining stiffness. A frame must therefore be both stable and stiff but yet not too hard in order to ensure a comfortable ride. The ride characteristics required depend on the intended use.

So what is the difference between bikes that look more or less similar?

Geometry

The frame geometry is the result of tube angle and length. The ride quality is determined by the head tube angle, which is 74 degrees for an all-round racing bike. A flatter angle of 73 degrees will give the bike better directional stability, making it a good long distance bike suitable for road races or tours. If the angle is greater though (75 degrees), the handlebar is more sensitive, making the bike more suited to circuit races but less so for tours. A shorter wheelbase (distance between the wheel axles) or about 100 cm makes a bike more maneuverable but also slightly less smooth compared to a longer, more comfortable wheelbase.

The fork also influences the ride comfort. The greater the pre-bend, the better the suspension. The rider looking for comfort should avoid very stiff and straight upright forks. A suspension fork increases the comfort, particularly on rough and poorly-surfaced roads.

The big manufacturers usually offer moderate geometries for all-round racing bikes with balanced ride qualities, so you don't need to think too much about this; however, test rides will reveal clear differences between the bikes.

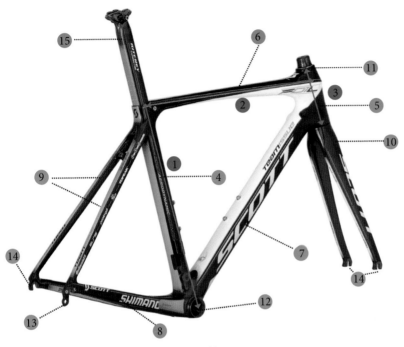

1. Seat tube length
2. Top tube length
3. Head tube length
4. Seat tube
5. Head tube
6. Top tube
7. Down tube
8. Chain stay
9. Seat stays
10. Fork (fork blades)
11. Head set
12. Bottom bracket shell
13. Derailleur hanger
14. Dropouts
15. Seat post

Fig. 10.1: A racing bike frame and its components

The **diamond frame** is the oldest and also the most tried and tested type of frame geometry. Despite numerous attempts with other frame shapes and different materials, the diamond frame is still the shape that will stand the test of time into the future. The diamond frame consists of 11 tubes formed into a triangle (rear triangle) and a quadrilateral (known as the main triangle although it actually has four sides). Diamond frames are characterized by a very high vertical stiffness and a significantly lower lateral stiffness—a problem that engineers have long been working on with only moderate success. However, the available lateral stiffness is usually sufficient and has improved considerably thanks to modern carbon technology.

Carbon, aluminum or steel?
In the lower and mid-price category, aluminum frames have completely replaced steel frames. There is now a wide variety of light, stable, and also still relatively cheap aluminum framed

bikes on the market. On the pro circuit, frames are almost exclusively carbon, and also in the cyclosportive and amateur scene, carbon frames also dominate in the higher price categories.

Steel

Steel has almost completely disappeared as a component of racing bike frames, and these frames are now only ridden by aficionados, although they are now undergoing a small renaissance. The main reason for the disappearance of steel frames is weight. Steel has high stability and sufficient resilience; however the specific weight at 7.86 gm/ dm3 is very high. Triple-butted (different wall thicknesses) tubes

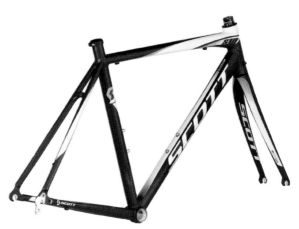

Fig. 10.2: Aluminum frames are light, strong, and cheap.

made of a chrome-molybdenum-steel alloy are normally used, with differing wall thicknesses and alloy compositions. Very thin wall thicknesses or 0.35 to 1 mm require the frame to be manufactured very carefully. However, steel frames quite justifiably have the reputation for being very durable and can last several decades. If they do get bent, it is very easy for a specialist to straighten them out again. Good paintwork, including primer, also stops any rust forming.

Aluminum

Aluminum is characterized by its low weight of 2.7 gm/dm3. However, as its strength is low, wall widths must be thicker and the diameter of the tubes greater, although this still makes the frame weight lower than that of a traditional steel one. Aluminum frames are welded and are available in many different geometries and quality grades. Here you should put your trust in the models of the big, well-known manufacturers, although less well-known brands also have good frames. That is because big factories in China and Taiwan build frames for many manufacturers at the same time and also provide technical highlights for no-name brands. This also applies to carbon frames.

Carbon

Carbon as a raw material is extremely resilient and has a very low specific weight of 1.75 gm/dm^3. However, the different carbon fibers must be combined with a resin which reduces their elasticity and increases their weight. Improvements in adhesive technologies (tube-to-tube process) and the adjustment of windings and layer thicknesses to stress now enable the manufacture of very good and extremely light frames, although they are significantly more expensive than aluminum frames. However, carbon frames do have one advantage—they are better at absorbing shock than other frames so are more comfortable. The bottom bracket and head tube stiffness obtained by carbon frames are also unrivaled. This, combined with their lightness, is the reason why carbon framed road-racing bikes are so popular.

Titanium

As a frame material, titanium is characterized by great strength and relatively low weight (4.5 kg/dm^3). The light and, in comparison to aluminum and carbon frames, rather soft titanium frames are very expensive and are only sold by a few manufacturers. From a technical point of view they are not an alternative to carbon.

Tip for beginners

Beginners are advised to buy a mid-priced aluminum frame.

Frame size

The right frame size is critical to get the right position on the bike. If you choose one that is much too small or large, you will not be able to set the bike up to fit you properly.

For decades, the frame size was only specified by the frame height. These days, the frame length (i.e., the top tube length) is equally important when it comes to choosing a frame.

Frame height

The frame height is either measured from the middle of the bottom bracket to the top of the seat tube or the top of the top tube (in Italy: to the center of the top tube). Nowadays, unlike in the days of steel frames, it is no longer possible to present a standardized table for frame sizes, because manufacturers' geometries and measuring methods are now too different.

In general, there is a trend toward smaller frames that are stiffer and lighter. Frame height is principally determined by leg length, so someone with shorter legs will choose a smaller frame.

Basically, you should be guided by the manufacturer's information and sizing recommendations. Descriptions from XS to XXL are often used, which tie in nicely with athletes' clothing sizes.

Women normally choose a frame about 1 to 2 cm smaller than men of the same height, as their upper body is often shorter in relation to their legs than men's. A frame bought according to leg length often proves to be too long. Youth cyclists are advised to buy a frame that is slightly too big to allow for growth. Tall and heavy riders (> 100 kg) are better off buying a more stable and therefore heavier frame and avoiding very light frames so that even a large frame will provide sufficient lateral stability and durability.

Frame length

As well as height, frame length is a key criterium for the right frame size. When purchasing a frame off the shelf, you have little control over the length; though, you can just choose between different brands, which may offer different lengths. Riders with extremely long or short upper bodies should get a bike made to measure, if they can't find a standard one that fits. However, by adjusting the length of the handlebar stem, you can get a bike with an otherwise unsuitable frame length to fit you.

10.2 Gear System

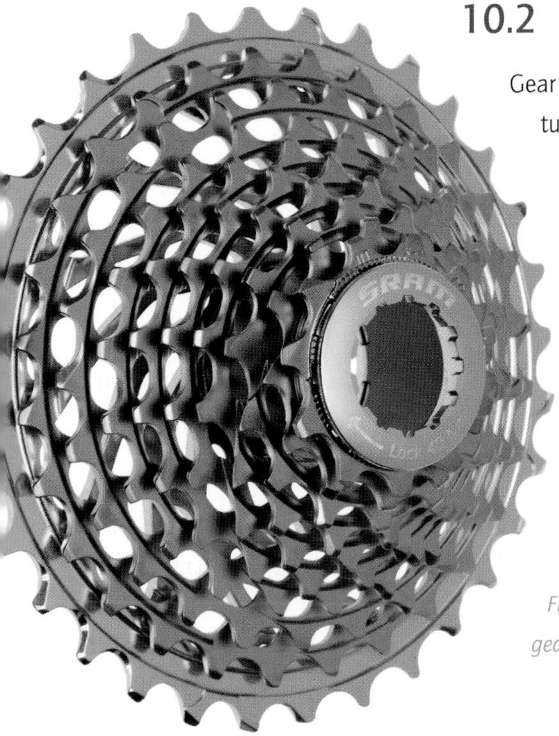

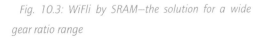

Gear systems are produced by three big manufacturers. Campagnolo is the oldest of the three with the longest tradition, Shimano is the one with the largest market share, and SRAM is the newcomer in the racing bike market, offering high-end and very functional racing bike group sets in different price categories. A few years ago, Shimano and Campagnolo introduced electronic gear systems that work fantastically well.

Fig. 10.3: WiFli by SRAM—the solution for a wide gear ratio range

Sprocket and chainwheel

The shifter adapts the gear ratio to different types of terrain and performance abilities. Due to the many innovations in recent years, shifting is now very easy, and 20 or even 22 gears (33 gears in triple chainwheels) are now common. Ten sprockets on the rear wheel are now standard, while Campagnolo provides eleven. With so many gears, the development range is well covered, and it is now possible to ride both steep climbs and also descents in a suitable gear ratio. Someone who cycles on the flat should choose a sprocket set with 12 to 21 or 23 cogs, while a mountain cyclist should choose one with 12 to 25 or 27 cogs. More reliable than triple chainwheels are compact cranks, which combine two smaller chainwheels. So instead of 53 and 39 cogs, we have chainwheels with 50 and 34 cogs and also an 11 to 27 cassette. With this gear ratio, even less fit cyclists can master long climbs. An even wider range is provided by the WiFli solution from SRAM, which contains a cassette with 11 to 32 cogs, although this requires a derailleur with a long cage.

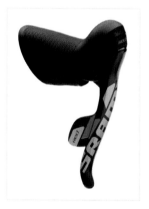

Fig. 10.4: Shifter: allows simultaneous control of both brakes and gears.

Shifter

The shifter allows safe, comfortable shifting and braking without the need to let go of the handlebar, which is much safer in all riding situations and particularly when racing. Whether you go for Campagnolo, SRAM, or Shimano components is ultimately a question of personal preference, as all three manufacturers have many advantages and disadvantages but all are very high quality. The manufacturer's shifters all work according to different logic. The one you choose after trying them out in the bike store is a question of taste, as the systems work very well, and professional races have been won with all three.

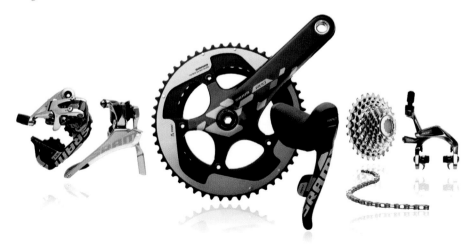

Front derailleur

The derailleur makes it possible to change the chain between the large and small chainwheels and is operated by the left brake lever. A small deflector, also called a chain spotter, stops the chain dropping down, which could lead to falls. Only when the derailleur is correctly set up does it work properly. This requires rather more experience and skill than when setting up a rear derailleur.

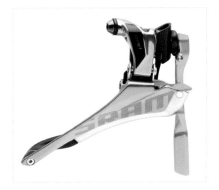

Fig. 10.5: The front derailleur moves the chain from the small chainwheel to the large one.

Rear derailleur

The rear derailleur has two change rollers which take care of the shifting process of the chain on the sprocket set. High-end rear derailleurs are now made of a material mix of carbon, aluminum, and titanium. A rear derailleur is not an expendable part—it just needs to be set up correctly.

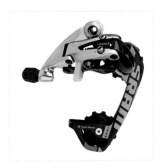

Chain

The chain transfers power from the pedal to the sprocket and, along with the tires, is the only expendable part of a racing bike, which must be changed regularly. The chain is subject to a great deal of wear and tear due to the forces acting on it and the dirt it is exposed to. After about 1,500 to 4,000 mi, depending on quality and usage even when it is well looked after, a chain needs replacing in order to avoid unnecessary wear on the other parts of the drive train.

Fig. 10.6: A very lightweight, high-end rear derailleur made of a material mix.

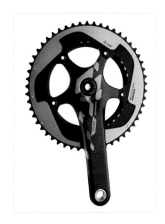

Cranks

Nowadays, pedal cranks and bottom brackets form a single unit in which the axel is firmly attached to the right crank. The left crank is screwed into the axel with a socket screw. The ball bearings are found in two bearing shells which are screwed into the frame (GXP Standard). In press-fit-brackets, a plastic casing with the ball bearings is pressed into the frame and also the axel. Gone are the days of complicated adjustments with expensive tools.

Fig. 10.7: Crank by SRAM with GXP bottom bracket

10.3 Brakes

Good brakes are an essential prerequisite for safe cycling. By law, a racing bike must have two brakes, one for each wheel. The braking system consists of a shifter attached to the handlebar; the brake cables and outer casing, which transfer the pull on the lever to the brakes; the brake calipers themselves; and finally the wheel rim on which the brake pads rub. The left brake lever operates the front wheel brake, which is responsible for two thirds of the total breaking effect. The right lever is responsible for the rear wheel. The outer casing (steel spirals with an inner plastic tubing) are always placed under the bar tape. In cycle racing, only side pull brakes, otherwise known as dual pivot brakes, are used, in which the leverage is more favorable due to the compact construction. A key criterium for brake quality is good modulation; a hard pull on the brakes should not make the wheels block suddenly which can cause a fall. Instead you should be able to carry on braking so that you can also perform sensitive braking maneuvers.

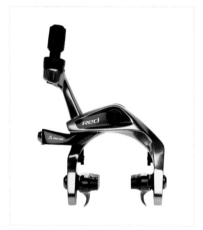

Fig. 10.8: The current generation of brakes tick almost all the boxes; precise and powerful braking with light hand pressure ensures safety.

Even the cheaper brakes produced by both big component manufacturers meet the these requirements and are definitely race-worthy.

Recently, racing bikes with disk brakes have also come onto the market, and it remains to be seen whether the disk brakes are as popular in road racing as they have been on mountain bikes. Experts are rather skeptical on this issue.

10.4 Wheels

A wheel in cycle racing terminology also includes the hub, spokes, rims, and tires. Wheels are a true technical miracle; their individual components may be very weak, but together they form a complex structure in the form of an extremely stable and also very light wheel. A good wheel can bear a weight of up to 500 kg without being permanently deformed. The high air pressure in the tires combined with the free movement of the hubs form the real secret of the smooth running of a racing bike. The hubs form the center of the wheel; they house the spoke heads and establish a connection with a frame. The smooth running depends primarily on the free movement of the hub bearing. In the most commonly used cone ball bearings, the ball bearings rotate between the two cones in a layer of grease. Lately, manufacturers have tended to produce hubs with industrial bearings that are completely maintenance-free and long-lasting. Such hubs are characterized by a silky-smooth, extremely low friction ride.

Each spoke is really weak in itself but as soon as they are under tension (preload), they are able to support enormous forces and carry the rider's bodyweight. A normal racing bike has 32 or 36 spokes, each one usually crossing three others. Pre-assembled wheel sets, known as *system wheels*, sometimes come with only 12 traditional or flat carbon spokes per wheel. However, these spokes are very highly pre-tensed, which makes for a very stable but also light and aerodynamic wheel. Often, these wheels are only recommended for riders weighing less than 176 lb. Two-millimeter-thick double-butted spokes predominate, whose central section has a diameter of 1.6 mm. The thinning in the center increases the resilience of the spokes so that they crack less easily. The critical point on a spoke is the curved head—the point where the spoke sits in the hub flange. This is where most spoke breaks occur. To improve the aerodynamics of the racing bike, bladed spokes are also used.

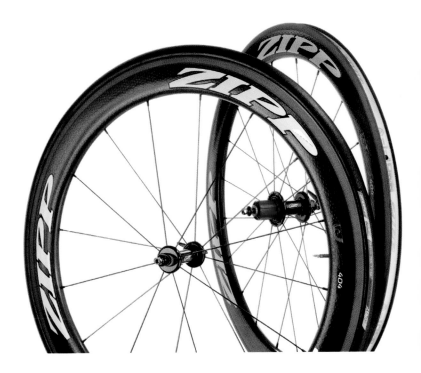

Fig. 10.9: If you like to ride fast and are riding in the mountains, you should make sure your wheels are light and also aerodynamic (Zipp 404 Firecrest).

A *rim* is defined as a metal bar bent into a circular shape, usually made of an aluminum alloy, which is usually joined to the *sidewall*. A cleanly-worked sidewall is essential for a high quality rim. The durability and stability of a rim is highly dependent on its weight and geometry (width, height, wall thickness). The optimal rim for mixed purposes is a hard-anodized, drop-shaped aluminum rim. The high vertical stiffness stops the rim from flattening as it rolls, which also considerably reduces the strain on the spokes so that they are much less inclined to break.

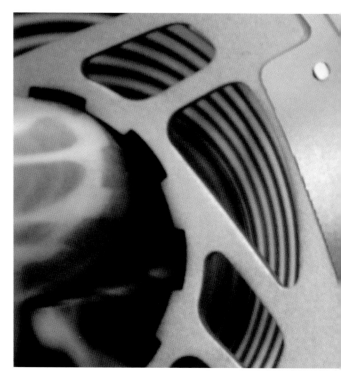

Carbon rims are much lighter than aluminum ones and can be flat and light or very high (up to 100 mm) and aerodynamic. It is also now possible to buy full-carbon rims for the practical wired-on tires. The absolute lightweights under the carbon rims are, however, produced for stuck-on tubular tires. The use in cobblestone races such as the Paris–Roubaix and cross-country races shows the impressive robustness of carbon rims. If you change your wheels frequently you must also change your brake pads, as special brake pads are required for carbon.

Purchasing Tip

If you like to ride fast, you should buy aerodynamic wheels with very high rims and few bladed spokes. Climbers prefer extremely light wheel sets, which are now produced by several manufacturers. Otherwise, 32-spoke wheels with industrially-mounted hubs and drop-shaped aluminum rims are very durable and smooth-running.

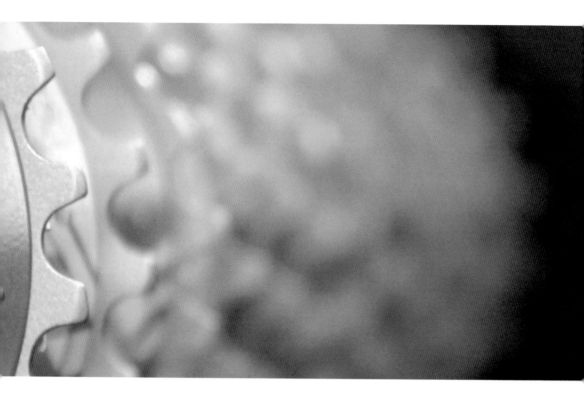

10.5 Tires

Racing cyclists are very superstitious when it comes to choosing their tires. Tires are the contact with the ground and what makes the difference between gripping or slipping. Cyclists who take part in races use very expensive tires that offer optimal road-holding combined with minimal rolling resistance. The narrower the tires, the poorer the grip and rolling resistance, but the lower the weight. So tire construction for manufacturers and tire choice for cyclists involves a considered comparison of different properties, for no tire is perfect for all conditions, and a compromise is necessary. For bicycle tourists, grip is less important, as they rarely take corners at top speed. Ride comfort and durability are what matters most. A mid-priced 23-mm tire is therefore the tire of choice for most cyclists. Usually, the top tires are very highly weight-optimized at the expense of running performance. A modern folding tire is prepared using dual or triple compound technology and has a low-wear surface and softer, better gripping sides for cornering. Underneath there is a third layer that reduces rolling resistance.

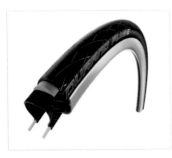

Fig. 10.10: A thick puncture protection belt provides long-term protection against punctures (Schwalbe Durano Plus).

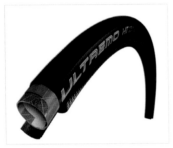

There are basically two different types of tires: tubular and folding, or wired-on/clincher tires. While tubular tires ("sew-ups") have a stitched-in inner tube and are stuck onto the rim, in folding or clincher tires, the tire and inner tube are separate. Clincher tires have a wire bead that interlocks with flanges in the rim. Tubular tires are currently experiencing a comeback due to the development of very light carbon rims. Only when combined with tubular tires can the wheel weight of carbon rims be significantly reduced. However, they have a range of disadvantages for recreational cyclists, such as the tedious and time-consuming gluing on of the tire, or the problem of changing tires after a puncture en route (for slight punctures you can use a sealer spray).

However, high-quality clinchers are also used by many racing cyclists in road and circuit races, particularly because they are much simpler to use and they offer better durability and value for money.

Fig. 10.11: Tubular tires are back in fashion due their light carbon rims. They roll extremely smoothly and have better running flat properties in the case of punctures (Schwalbe Ultremo HT).

Purchasing Tip
- The rubber compound of the running surface should be grippy but robust (road grip).
- If possible, use 23 mm or 25 mm tires; they provide enough ride comfort, have low rolling resistance and grip and very rarely puncture.
- Try to buy light tires (around 200 g).
- Profile is less important; if the rubber compound is correct, slicks (smooth-tread tires) can even be used in the rain.

As far as tire pressure is concerned, you should follow manufacturers' guidelines, which are printed on the side of the tire. The general rule is that extremely high tire pressure should only be used when low rolling resistance is required (time trials, races). Otherwise, you should allow a more comfortable ride for your back and joints and pump up your tires moderately (7 bars). They will still roll smoothly enough like this. The fact is, though, that most riders train with too little air pressure, which leads to punctures that could have been avoided.

10.6 Saddle

The racing saddle is one of three points of contact between rider and bike. It supports considerably less bodyweight than the handlebar, and in the case of frequent cycling, regularly leads to seat problems.

In cycle racing, narrow saddles with very slim noses are used, which prevents the thigh from rubbing against the saddle. Saddle frames made of steel, titanium, or carbon are spread over the base like a tent. As plastic saddles do not need to be broken in and are less damaged by rain, nowadays almost all saddles are made of plastic with a leather or plastic cover. Depending on the model, padded layers are found above the plastic base of the saddle (some manufacturers also use gel inserts). Also available are extremely light saddles weighing around 100 g with no padding at all. However, this lightness is usually combined with a significant loss of comfort.

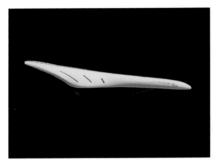

Fig. 10.12: Despite its extreme lightness, the Arione by Fizik is a comfortable saddle with a carbon frame and base.

A saddle should not be too soft or have too much padding, as in the long run, harder saddles are more comfortable. Anatomically-shaped saddles have special padding for the sit bones and a groove for the urethra. Saddles with holes in the middle are also very popular with some cyclists. Also available are shorter, slightly wider saddles that meet the requirements of female anatomy; however they are only rarely used by top female cyclists.

Purchasing Tip

In the end, it takes a few attempts to find your ideal saddle that you no longer need to change. A suspension seat post can provide a much more comfortable ride.

10.7 Handlebar

Drop handlebars offer several possible ergonomic grip positions: on top near the stem (tops), on the hooks (on the top bend), on the brakes (hoods), on the lower part of the bar (drops), or simply on the ends of the bar. This was not always the case, as the first drop handlebars could only be held on the drops.

Drop handlebars weigh between 200 and 350 g with widths varying from 36 to 46 cm. Men of average height require a 40 to 44 cm handlebar, while a 38 cm one is best for women. As a guide, handlebar width should roughly correspond to shoulder width. The ends of the handlebars must be covered, as otherwise the sharp ends of the bars could cause serious injuries in the event of a fall.

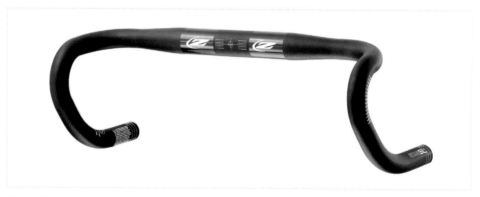

Fig. 10.13: Drop handlebars should be anatomically shaped. Flat or wide sections on the top of the bar considerably improve ride comfort.

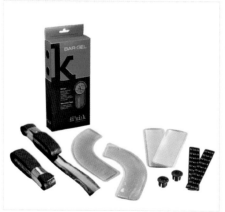

Bar tape

Drop handlebars are wrapped with bar tape, which should be non-slip, able to absorb sweat, and slightly padded. Gel pads under the tape ensure better pressure distribution and a larger handlebar diameter that affords better grip.

Fig. 10.14: Grippy bar tape and gel pads by Fizik.

10.8 Pedal Systems

Since the pedal revolution launched by the firm Look and Bernard Hinault in 1985, clipless pedals have continued to evolve, but the basic principle has remained the same. Then only produced by one manufacturer, now many firms offer their own different pedal systems. All modern pedals are based on the safety pedal in which the rider's foot must automatically be released in the event of a fall in order to avoid serious injury. They should also be as easy to put on and take off as possible.

An adaptor under the shoe slots into a recess in the pedal by means of a locking mechanism. A twisting action of the foot releases the lock. The formerly standard, absolutely rigid pedal-shoe connections prevent the natural rotational movement of the lower leg during the pedaling action, possibly leading to knee and other joint problems.

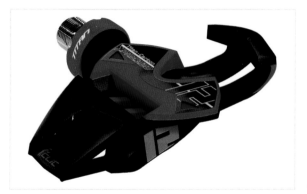

The lighter the pedals and shoes, the lower the mechanical effort required to move their weight.

Fig. 10.15: The time system is particularly ergonomic (easy on the joints and tendons).

The firm Time has developed a pedal system that allows the foot the necessary freedom of movement. Many pros prefer this system. The pedal is only released when the foot exceeds a certain angle of rotation (5 degrees on each side). This anatomically sound idea has gradually been adopted by other manufacturers, such as Look, Shimano, and Speedplay.

Purchasing Tip

Cyclists with orthopedic leg problems should use a pedal system with lateral freedom of movement for the feet and the smallest possible gap between the sole of the foot and the pedal.

10.9 Accessories

A bike computer can be used to record and manage training. It shows the mileage covered, speed, training time, and other useful data for training and racing that can be transferred to your training diary at home.

Top models allow data to be stored and consulted later. It can also be evaluated using analysis software.

If possible, choose a user-friendly computer that shows two or more pieces of data at the same time.

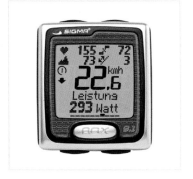

Fig. 10.16: The Sigma Rox stores all recorded information. It can then be evaluated using analysis software.

Mini pump

You should always take a mini pump with you on training rides, along with a spare inner tube and a repair kit. When choosing a mini pump, go for a stable model that allows for high pressure. An extendable tube makes pumping easier and reduces the risk of damaging the valve. A universal valve head can also be used for Schrader or American valves.

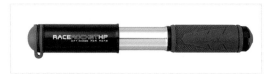

Fig. 10.17: A mini pump like the Racerocket is an invaluable aid in the event of a puncture, as 8 bar are no problem for these little guys.

Floor pump

A floor pump allows you to fill a tire quickly and effortlessly to the correct air pressure, which is why it is an ideal pump to use at home. The pump should look stable, have an ergonomic grip, and must have a pressure display. A multi-valve head on a long tube allows you to pump up inner tubes with different types of valves, and add-on valves even allow you to pump up balls or inflatable mattresses. The pump is fixed to the floor by standing on the feet.

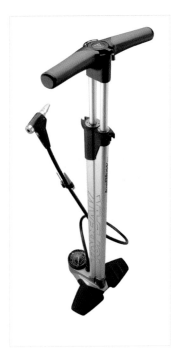

Fig. 10.18: A floor pump like the Joe Blow Ace is perfect for home use.

Tools

Ninety-five percent of all small repair jobs can be carried out en route with a multifunction tool kit comprising an Allen key set, screwdriver, and various ring spanners. A chain riveting tool, spoke wrench, and a small pair of pliers make more complicated repairs possible and could even occasionally repair the tools at home, but you should learn how to use them first as their wide range of functions can make them tricky to use. At only 100 to 300 g, mini tools are extremely light and fit into any jersey or in the saddle bags.

Caution is required, though, when it comes to buying cheap tools from a discount store, as the quality is usually only average, which can lead to rounded Allen screws.

Your workshop should also be equipped with high quality tools. If you just do occasional repairs, the following list is all you need;

- Good Allen key (2-10 mm)
- Wire cutter
- Universal pliers
- Phillips screwdriver
- Spoke wrench
- Chain riveter
- Open-ended spanner (8-15)
- Sprocket remover
- Chain whip
- Chain oil, penetrating oil spray, ball bearing grease, rags

If you regularly assemble entire bikes, the prepstation by Topeak is recommended.

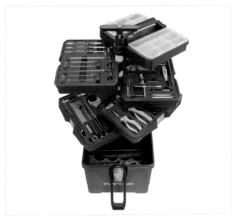

Fig. 10.19: The prepstation by Topeak contains all the tools you need to assemble a bike in a compact format and has wheels to make it portable. A mobile workstation that is not just for professional teams.

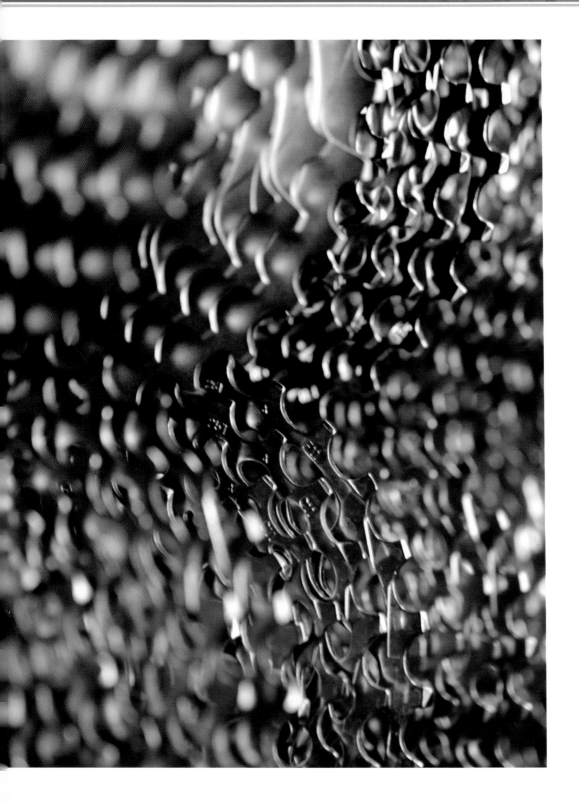

Assembly stands

If you tinker with your bike more regularly, you would benefit from being able to hang your bike comfortably from an assembly stand. It is important to look for a secure, universal quick-release clamp for frame tubes of different thicknesses that folds down into a compact size.

Mudguards

Particularly in the winter months, road cyclists have to contend with wet roads. Clip-on mudguards are an ideal way to help you to stay clean and dry during training. It is important to be able to put them on and take them off quikkly, and they should be vibration-free and securely fastened. Stick adhesive film over the frame under the clip to avoid scratching the paintwork.

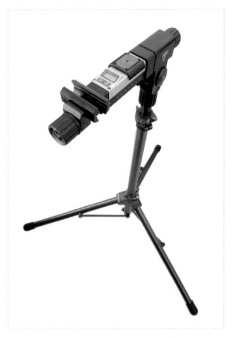

Fig. 10:20: An assembly stand with a built-in weighing scale should be part of every workshop (Topeak prepstand Elite Pro).

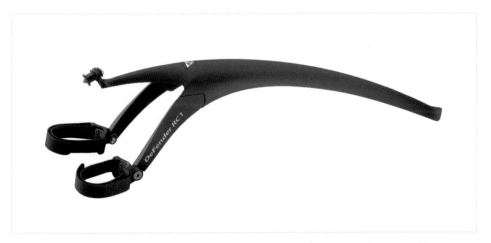

Fig. 10.21: Clip-on mudguards increase the possible training time in winter and spring and keep the cyclist dry and healthy (Topeak Defender).

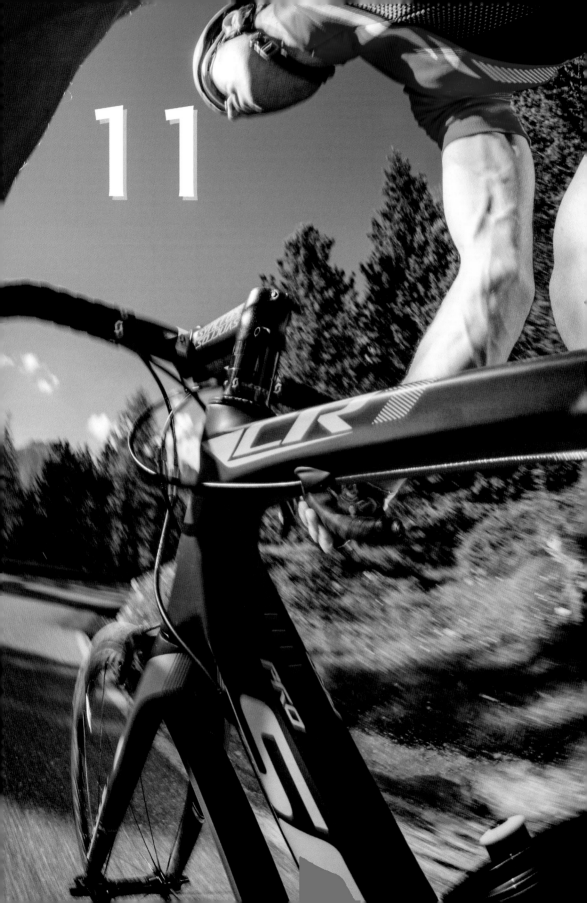

11. Functional Clothing

High quality functional clothing is essential for cycling to be really enjoyable, as this is the only way to protect the body effectively, especially from the weather. In recent years, the functional cycling clothing available on the market has increased dramatically. The most important features of different garments are described below.

The layering principle

Basically, you should dress for training according to the layering principle. Several thin layers with different functions guarantee an optimal skin climate and the necessary protection from weather conditions. In addition, the individual layers are very thin and light thanks to modern technology and are therefore very comfortable to wear. If one layer is no longer required, you can just take it off and pop it into your jersey pocket (e.g., windproof gilet or arm warmers).

Cyclists tend to wear rather figure-hugging, tight clothing. Racing cyclists even tend to wear a jersey a size smaller than normal. Bike tourists on the other hand prefer a looser fit. The benefit of functional clothing is greatest when it is worn directly against the skin without an additional air cushion.

11.1 Underwear

Nothing feels more uncomfortable than a sweaty cotton undershirt that feels cold and sticky on your skin and even feels freezing cold on a descent. Irrespective of external temperatures, cyclists should therefore always wear a functional undershirt directly next to the skin. Unlike cotton, synthetic fibers absorb very little moisture. The special structure of the weave wicks sweat away from the skin into the next layer of clothing, thus keeping the skin considerably drier than other types of undershirt, which means a higher skin temperature and reduced loss of warmth and therefore energy. Particularly in cold weather, the functional undershirt always feels warm and dry. Only when temperatures hit 86 °F do some cyclists dispense with the functional undershirt, but also only when no long descents are planned. In hot weather, a functional undershirt is not uncomfortable and also feels much nicer against the skin than a jersey.

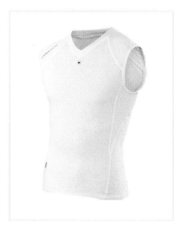

Fig. 11.1: A functional undershirt is just as important as your jersey and should not be scrimped on. Cotton absorbs more than 10 times as much moisture as special functional materials.

Polyamide or polyester is the material used. All weave patterns are based on a network structure. We find coarsely woven undershirts and only apparently denser and thicker materials. Sometimes the materials used by some manufacturers tend to take on a musty odor. You can investigate this on the Internet.

A good functional undershirt costs between $30 and $60, which is definitely worth it and will be repaid by a few less days off training due to head colds.

Functional undershirts can be bought with no sleeves, with short and long sleeves, or with or without roll necks. They can also be purchased with a sewn-on, windproof layer of material, known as a windbreaker. These undershirts are recommended for riding in the mountains and in winter.

Cellular shirts are highly recommended, as they allow a lot of air onto the skin and keep you amazingly warm. Another advantage of functional undershirts is their ability to dry quickly after a quick wash in the washer.

In cold temperatures, more densely and thickly woven thermal undershirts may be worn. An insulating intermediate layer made of thin fleece or other thermal material is also advisable when the temperature drops below zero.

11.2 Jersey

The jersey is the next layer on top of the undershirt. Thirty years ago, they were usually still made of cotton, but now jerseys are made of different synthetic fabrics. They are therefore only able to absorb a little sweat and do not get soaked with moisture. Thick jersey fabrics, sometimes with a fleecy interior, are intended for use on cooler days and thinner materials are suitable for hot days. Zip-up jerseys provide the necessary wind cooling during climbs on hot days, but also risk trapping insects.

A good fit is also important; the back in particular should not be too short in order to provide sufficient protection for the kidneys. A jersey should be close-fitting and not flap about in the wind. Sewn-in pockets on the back provide storage space for a rain jacket, cell phone, spare inner tube, pump, and energy bars.

For cooler days, long-sleeved jerseys may be worn, also with long zips as jersey jackets.

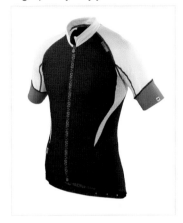

11.3 Cycling Shorts

Cycling shorts differ from other sports shorts due to a sewn-in chamois leather lining or seat cushion that is still called leather even though it is now made of easy-care synthetic material. The seat cushion prevents chafing of the seat area, cushions it somewhat, and protects from cold. This happens by means of a terry-toweling insert in the front part.

Fig. 11.2: Jerseys should be tight-fitting and be made of breathable material.

Cycling shorts should be tight-fitting and not wrinkle or pinch. Shorts with a bib are always preferable to those without as they provide better coverage of the kidneys and therefore protect them from the cold and just fit better. However, bib shorts present a problem for women when they need to answer the call of nature quickly. But tights with quick release fasteners on the bibs are now available. Tights made of six or eight anatomically cut panels fit better than one made of only four panels of material.

Cycling shorts should be washed after every training session to stop germs in the seat pad rubbing into the skin, which would lead to saddle sores.

In cooler weather, you can wear three-quarter length and long tights, also with bibs and seat pads. Long tights are usually made of thicker, fleece-lined material, which sometimes have windproof but also flexible patches on the knees or the whole of the front.

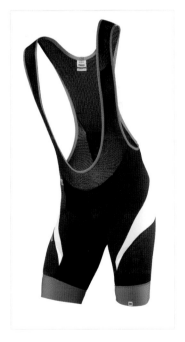

Fig. 11.3: Shorts are the cyclist's most important item of clothing.

11.4 Useful Accessories

Cycling gloves

Originally conceived as brake gloves for the track, cycling gloves have a different function in road cycling. They pad the hard handlebar to stop blisters forming on the palms of the hands when cycling on poor road surfaces. They also protect the hands from abrasions in the event of a fall, which is particularly important in road races due to the increased risk of falling. Gloves improve the grip on the handlebar in wet weather. When buying gloves, look for a good fit and synthetic leather, as gloves that are too big will wrinkle and cause pressure points and blisters.

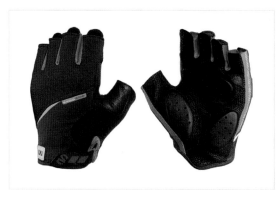

Fig. 11.4: Cycling gloves cushion the hands against vibrations and stop pressure points and numb fingers.

Arm warmers, knee warmers, and leg warmers

In transitional seasons, on a still cold summer morning or a cool day, arm and leg warmers can be used; they are special sleeves or trouser legs that are worn underneath the jersey or tights. Leg and arm warmers can be made of various different types of material. Thermal leg warmers can be worn into late fall as protection against the cold.

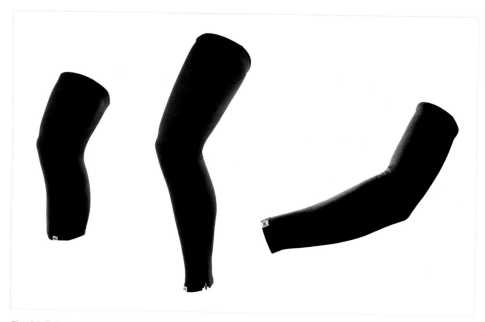

Fig. 11.5: Leg warmers are sufficient at temperatures down to about 47 °F. For cool summer days, knee warmers are ideal.

Rain jacket

No cyclist should leave home without a rain jacket, as they are not only useful during wet rides or sudden showers, but can also be worn on long descents or when returning from a tour in the evening to keep the cold at bay. The rain jacket should have a Velcro or zip fastener and be longer at the back to protect against spray water. Rain jackets are cut very short in the front so that they don't wrinkle up. Low quality rain jackets are made of waterproof and airtight material, while high quality ones are waterproof but also breathable fabrics. A rain jacket should be close-fitting and not flap about in the airflow.

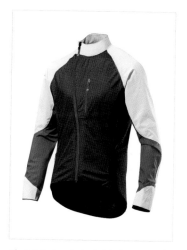

Fig 11.6: A rain jacket is longer at the back than the front to stop the seat getting wet, while breathable side panels allow air to circulate.

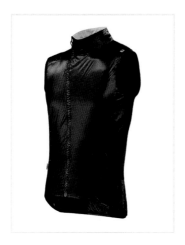

Fig. 11.7: A wind vest fits under any jersey and keeps you warm.

Wind bib

A wind bib is a sleeveless garment that is worn in front of the chest under the jersey to protect from the wind. The front is made of windproof material while the back can be made of normal material. Functional undershirts with windproof fronts are also available.

Wind vest

If the weather is definitely rain-free, then a wind vest (without sleeves) is a very useful item of clothing for descents or when riding in the cold. Also after hard training, the vest stops the wet skin from cooling down.

One-piece race suit

One-pieces are often worn for circuit races in the summer; they are skin-tight and made of very thin material. Their advantage is that they are very aerodynamic and allow sweat to evaporate. They are not suitable for touring cyclists and for training purposes though as they usually have no pockets, and they do not keep you warm during rest breaks.

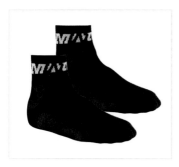

Fig. 11.8: The length of racing socks has decreased dramatically in recent years, and colored or even black ones are now available.

Socks

Every cyclist's wardrobe should also include special socks that are very short and often still white. Made of Coolmax, they keep your feet dry and at the right temperature. You can always tell immediately what kind of cyclist someone is by their socks. In racing circles, tennis socks or even knee-length socks are considered to be very uncool.

11.5 Winter Clothing

Cyclists who train year-round need warm cycling apparel for the fall and spring but most of all for winter. With the right clothing, you can even cycle in temperatures around freezing as long as the roads are free from snow and ice.

Thermal tights

At low temperatures, thermal tights keep the muscles and joints warm. The material is thicker and has a fleecy lining, providing a good layer of insulation against the cold and wind. An integrated wind protection for the knees is also recommended.

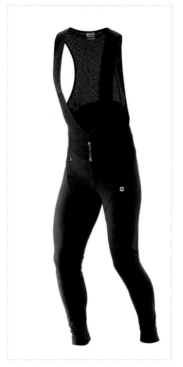

Fig. 11.9: Winter tights are made of different materials. Wind stopper material on the knees and thighs minimizes the loss of heat.

Winter jacket

Winter jackets are available in different temperature ratings. They range from a simple jersey jacket made of thick, fleecy thermal fabric that can comfortably be worn down to temperatures of around 50°F, to special jackets for temperatures below freezing. These are mainly composed of a padded jersey fabric with sewn-on windproof material on the front and sleeves. Very popular, too, is a kind of soft shell material that keeps out the air flow and is also warmer thanks to the thickness of the material. A fleecy lining and a high, close-fitting collar also keep your body warm even on cold days.

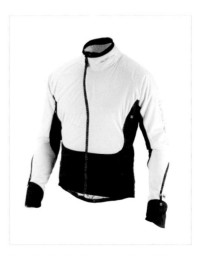

Fig. 11.10: A winter jacket must have a high, warm collar.

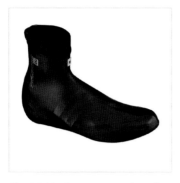

Overshoes

Neoprene overshoes protect the shoes and feet from getting cold, wet, and dirty. Neoprene has clear advantages over other materials: It is waterproof, insulating, durable, and easily washable. Special thin rain overshoes are used when racing in the rain in the summer, which keep the feet warm and relatively dry.

Fig. 11.11: Neoprene overshoes keep your feet warm even in the wet.

Tip

A low-cost alternative to often-pricey overshoes is to wear socks over your shoes with a hole cut in for the cleat. Even pros ride like this as feet sweat less in socks. In order to protect your feet from cold winds, you can also pull a thin freezer bag under your socks.

Thermal gloves

Thermal gloves made of different materials are also available. The important thing is that they are flexible enough to be able to grip the handlebar, which is not the case with thick downhill skiing gloves. Cross-country gloves are ideally suited to cycling, as long as it is not too cold. Special cycling gloves with a windproof layer are thin but still very warm.

Winter hat

It is advisable to wear a warm hat in the winter to protect the head, ears, and forehead from the often unpleasant cold air flow. It should be made from breathable material. As you also need to wear a helmet in winter, why not wear an under helmet hat, which, as the name suggests, can be worn underneath the helmet to keep the head warm and protect from the air flow. If this makes the helmet too tight, just remove one or more inner cushions.

11.6 The Right Clothes for Any Weather

The ideal clothing for different weather conditions is listed below:

> 86 °F	Functional undershirt, jersey (zip-up), cycling tights (cycling socks), helmet
77-86 °F	Functional undershirt, jersey (zip-up), cycling tights, cycling socks, helmet
68-77 °F	Functional undershirt, possibly with windbreaker or wind bib, jersey, cycling tights, helmet
59-68 °F	Functional undershirt, with windbreaker or wind bib, jersey with arm warmers or long-sleeved jersey, cycling tights with knee or leg warmers, wind vest, cycling socks, helmet
50-59 °F	Functional undershirt, with windbreaker or wind bib, jersey and long-sleeved jersey, cycling tights with leg warmers or long tights, wind vest, cycling socks, helmet (long gloves)
41-50 °F	Functional undershirt (long-sleeved), with windbreaker or wind bib, winter jacket and jersey, winter tights, long socks, overshoes, helmet, winter gloves
32-41 °F	Functional undershirt (long-sleeved), with windbreaker or wind bib, winter jacket and possibly turtleneck sweater, wind jacket, winter tights, warm knee socks, overshoes, helmet, under helmet hat with ear warmers, winter gloves
- 23-32 °F	Functional undershirt (long-sleeved), with windbreaker or wind bib, winter jacket and turtleneck sweater and possibly long-sleeved jersey, winter jacket, winter tights, knee warmers, warm knee socks, overshoes, helmet, under helmet hat with ear warmers, face mask, winter gloves
< 23 °F	See above. Training at these temperatures should not exceed 1.5 hours

Fig. 11.12: Weather/clothing table

Rain

Experienced cyclists are usually pretty good at predicting the weather and only take a rain jacket along if it looks like rain. Beginners should always tuck a small, folding rain jacket in their jersey pocket, as an hour's ride home in the rain at an unexpectedly cold 50 °F can lead to a serious respiratory tract infection.

Basic equipment

Basic equipment for those cyclists who would like to train mainly in the spring and summer and on warm fall days comprises the following items of clothing:

Functional undershirt, with windbreaker ($50) or wind bib, jersey ($90) with arm warmers ($30), cycling shorts ($100) with knee or leg warmers ($40), wind vest ($60), cycling socks ($15), helmet ($120).

It is hard to give prices for individual items of clothing, as they can vary greatly depending on manufacturer and quality. The prices given are approximates for mid-priced products.

For winter temperatures down to about 32 °F, you also need a winter jacket ($150), winter tights ($120), as well as overshoes ($40), and gloves ($40). Below 32 °F, bicycle racing is no longer very enjoyable for most cyclists.

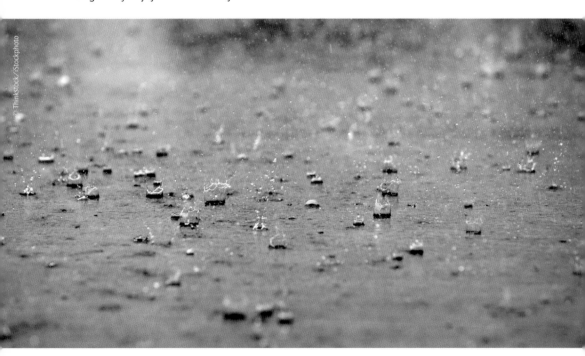

© ThinkStock/iStockphoto

11.7 Cycling Shoes

Cycling shoes make riding a bike more enjoyable and also make the transfer of power more economical, which is why you should not scrimp on shoes. Good cycling shoes have a stiff sole, usually made of plastic or carbon, in order to optimize the transfer of power from the foot to the pedal.

The uppers are often made of synthetic leather (dries quickly) or high-quality natural leather, combined with different synthetic mesh inserts for ventilation purposes. Velcro, twist-out, and ratchet fastenings have completely replaced laces in cycling shoes.

A cleat is fitted under the sole that clips into the pedal, which enables an economical pedaling action. The combination of stiff sole and cleat mean that these shoes are not exactly great for walking in; walking is actually difficult and damages the shoes. Nearly all shoes are now compatible with all modern pedal plates as cleats with three holes in the sole are now standard for most manufacturers.

Racing shoes must fit a little more snugly than normal shoes so that they have good stability when pushing and pulling on the pedal. The shoes should not be so tight that pressure points, particularly on the toes and toenails, form, though.

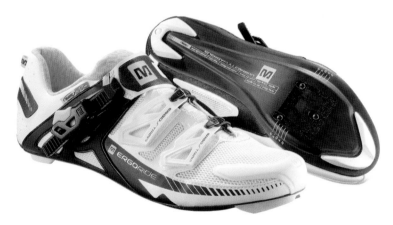

Fig. 11.13: Stiff soles, practical, adjustable lacing, and lightweight are the features of modern cycling shoes.

11.8 Helmet

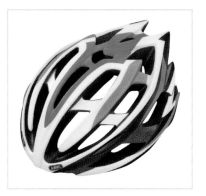

A helmet must be worn to protect you from serious injury. Most serious head injuries sustained in cycling accidents can be avoided by wearing a hard hat. It should fit snugly but not pinch and should have sufficient air vents.

The straps must be correctly adjusted and should not be loose-fitting so that the helmet does not just slip off your head in the event of an accident. Brightly-colored helmets are more visible in traffic.

Fig. 11.14: A cycling helmet is just as important as your bike, and it is negligent to ride without it.

A good helmet is available in several sizes, can be adjusted in a number of positions, and has cleverly-designed ventilation. Immolding helmets are the most robust and provide more protection than traditional ones in which the hard shell is stuck onto the helmet. For this reason, immolding helmets are also slightly more expensive. They should weigh less than 10.5 ounces.

In rain or when the sun is low in the sky, you can wear a racing cap under your helmet to improve visibility. For winter you can wear a very thin but still warm skull cap with ear warmers underneath your helmet.

Tip
The pads inside the helmet can be removed and carefully washed. The straps should also be washed occasionally. You must replace your helmet if you fall on your head, as hairline cracks stop the all-important energy absorption by the helmet material in the event of another fall.

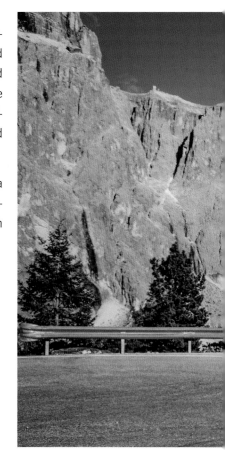

Cycling glasses

Wearing glasses for training and racing has several benefits for your eyes. They protect your eyes from the significant air flows associated with high speed, keep insects out of your eyes, and they cut out damaging UV radiation. In the event of a fall, glasses protect your eyes from injuries. Glasses, therefore, have a protective role and are not a fashion item, although they can still look good! As well as tinted glasses for sunny weather, you can also buy non-tinted or even brightening glasses for dull days. Glasses with interchangeable or light-adaptive lenses are recommended.

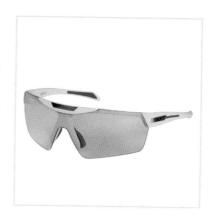

Fig. 11.15: Cycling glasses should not only look good but must also be functional and protect the eyes.

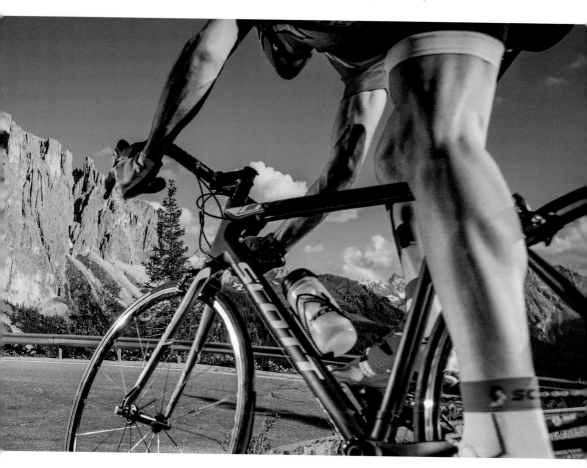

Glossary

Acid tolerance	Ability to tolerate high lactic acid concentrations (pain) in the blood.
Adaptation	The way the body changes as a result of training.
Aerobic energy release	Metabolic process that requires the presence of oxygen.
Anaerobic energy release	Metabolic process that does not require oxygen.
Belgian tourniquet	Rotating paceline, mainly in races, in which all riders up to the leader are able to benefit from the slipstream.
Citric acid cycle	Enzyme system of the energy metabolism that takes place in the mitochondria.
Concentric	Muscle activation that increases tension on a muscle as it shortens.
Contraction	Muscle tension.
Dehydration	Loss of water from the body when cycling with associated performance deterioration.
Dynamic	A muscle works dynamically when it moves a joint or performs physical work (opposite: static).
Eccentric	A yielding movement in which the muscles lengthen as they contract.
Echelon	Mainly formed during road races on the side of the road downwind, for the riders lined up behind each other the slipstream is reduced.
Enzyme	A protein that accelerates a metabolic reaction, many known ones exist.
Glycogen	Stored form of carbohydrates in the body (complex sugar, animal starch).
Intensity	Measure of training load, monitored by heart rate and feel.
Lactate	Lactic acid, metabolite of the anaerobic–lactate energy release, accumulates during high-intensity effort, causes muscle fatigue.
Macrocycle	Periodization cycle lasting from 4-8 weeks.
Maximal heart rate	Highest possible heart rate at maximum exertion.
Maximal oxygen consumption	Highest possible oxygen consumption of the body at maximum exertion.
Metabolism	All of the chemical processes to which endogenous substances and nutrients are subject.
Microcycle	Weekly training plan.

Microtrauma	The smallest injury.
Mitochondrion	The cell's power producers.
Mobilization	Excitement (mental).
Monosaccharide	Building block of complex carbohydrates, absorbed in the small intestine without being eliminated.
Muscle contraction	Shortening of a muscle.
Muscular imbalance	Imbalance between two muscles or muscle groups (e.g., between abdominal and back muscles).
Peloton	Field of cyclists.
Periodization	Division of the training year into several sections in order to build up and maintain certain conditioning abilities.
Polysaccharide	Carbohydrate (like glucose) composed of monosaccharides, must be split before being absorbed.
Recovery	Rest, physical recuperation, important for the training process.
Rehabilitation	Restoration of health following illness or injury.
Repetition	Number of times a movement is repeated per set in interval and strength training
Resting heart rate	The lowest heart rate at complete rest, usually in the morning.
Set	Way of measuring training volume in interval and strength training; a set consists of a number of repetitions.
Sport damage	To cause damage to a structure by repeated excessive stimuli.
Sports injury	An injury caused by a sudden external force.
Sprocket	Rear wheel gear rim.
Static	Without external movement, joint angles do not change.
Steady state	A state of equilibrium.
Visualization	Imaging a movement sequence in the context of a mental training program.
Volume	Training volume is measured in terms of mileage or training time.

Index

Photo Credits

Photos and graphics:

Abus: 314

Achim Schmidt: 12, 39, 44, 68, 76, 77, 113, 123-130, 132, 140, 155, 167-172, 174, 194, 195, 224, 226, 227, 228, 231, 232, 235, 238, 239, 241, 244, 247, 248, 252, 256, 260, 263, 264, 266, 275, 280, 286-303, 306-309, 312, 315, 316, 317

Centurion: 34, 40, 98

Comsport/Tino Pohlmann: 136, 144

Fizik: 295-296

Hennes Roth: 3, 10, 15, 18, 26, 41, 118, 121, 122, 147, 148, 157, 164, 166, 170, 179, 189, 190, 201, 202, 209, 219, 222, 242, 245, 261, 262, 268, 271, 278

Mavic: 304-310, 313

Tim de Waele/tdwsport.com (Scott): 3, 9, 25, 38, 43, 45, 53, 54, 55, 71, 135, 175, 206, 214, 221, 225, 254, 258, 269, 277

Topeak: 298-301

Schwalbe: 294

Scott: 16, 19, 131, 230, 284, 285, 315

Sigmasport: 66, 253

SRAM: 81, 111, 196, 229, 257, 282, 283, 287-293

Upsolut: 13

Team Multivan Merida: 123-130, 132

Layout:	Andrea Brücher
Typesetting:	Andreas Reuel
Coverdesign:	Sabine Groten
Coverphoto:	Tim de Waele With the kind permission of Scott Sports AG Germany

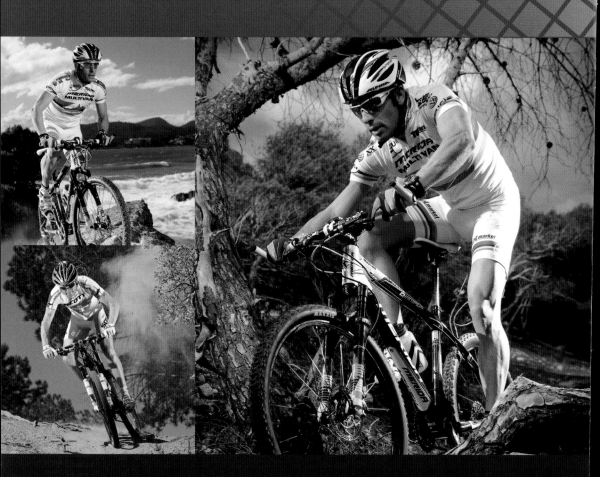

ACHIM SCHMIDT

MOUNTAIN BIKE
TRAINING

_TRAINING SCHEDULES FOR THE WHOLE YEAR
_**OPTIMIZED TRAINING MANAGEMENT**
_STRENGTH & MENTAL TRAINING

MEYER
& MEYER
SPORT

6 Training Management

6.1 Be Your Own Coach

"Be your own coach" is an American phrase, which is typical of the American approach to sport, particularly endurance sport. You are in the best position to know your body, feel the exhaustion, the strength and are also best placed to decide what is right for you in terms of training. However, a certain amount of knowledge is still required for this, which this book and others like it attempt to provide. It goes without saying that if you are lucky enough to have a good coach, you should be pleased and certainly not trying to get rid of him! Two heads are better than one, and by actively participating in the training planning and structuring with your coach you will achieve more, and the collaboration will be more successful. Absolute novices would find it hard alone and should seek the collaboration of experienced mountain bikers or coaches and then gradually work out their own idea of a structured training plan.

A sensible, self-constructed training plan based on a few important training rules guarantees good performance development. It is up to you to determine a sensible proportion of flexibility and highly structured training in order to be successful while also having fun. Solemnly and unthinkingly sticking 100% to a rigid program cannot achieve this. Listen to your body and decide what works for you and what doesn't. If you don't feel good after training or racing, rest for a day.

6.2 Your Own Training Plan

Now for a description of the procedure involved in drawing up a training plan according to the important principles of time management. First, the division of the phases should be examined in more detail. If you are preparing a training plan for the first time, you should allow yourself time to do it and, above all, obtain the advice of experienced mountain bikers in order to avoid possible mistakes. Often, novices and, in particular, ambitious athletes tend to overestimate their time budget, their motivation and their ability to recuperate. They make plans they cannot stick to, which may result in a completely incorrect build-up, low performance level and possibly a state of overtraining.

The opinion that only one training plan or one method can lead to elite level performance is fortunately mistaken. Different training methods lead to the goal, for everyone reacts differently to the training content, hence the importance of experimenting with different methods. What works for one cyclist does not necessarily work for another.

Reaching peak performance not only involves planning and executing training but also adjusting it. So while there are many different ways of preparing for success, amendments to the training plan are required in almost every case. Performance is consolidated and optimized with respect to the season's goal through systematic periodization and cyclization of intensity and volume.

If a training error is identified and rectified immediately, nothing is lost, but if training errors or poor performance are ignored, it is usually impossible to reach the goal you have set for the season.

Analysis of the Previous Year

Training planning also involves an analysis of the previous year. Many training errors can be identified using the notes in your training diary. These errors must definitely be addressed when preparing the new training plan and should be kept in mind in the following season, especially in the case of poor form. Tips for analyzing the previous year can be found in chapter 6.4.

Planning From Year to Year

When preparing your training plan, you need to take into account not just the preceding and coming years but also your long-term development. A continuous improvement in performance due to moderate increases in training is much better and also leads to less frequent drops in form and injuries than excessive increases in the annual training volume. Unstable performances can often be observed in the case of young amateurs, who do not yet have a solid foundation of endurance training. The annual training volume is measured in hours, of which a high proportion (about 60%) should be **BE 1** training.

The principle of continuous workload increase involves increases of, at most, approximately 15% at elite level. Higher loading increases of over 20% to about 40% are only possible in mountain biking at regional level. Only beginners are allowed to double their total training volume the following year, if appropriate. The higher the performance level, the more gradual the planned loading increases. Rehab bikers and beginners should be cautious, though, for physical exercise must be approached very gradually in order to avoid possible health risks.

Top cyclists who decide to stop competing at elite level should never reduce their training by more than 50% from one year to the next in order to eliminate any health risks. In the former GDR, endurance athletes at the end of the career were given training plans that reduced their training workload gradually. A basic training workload of about 200–250 hours per year should, however, be maintained in any case.

This is how it's done:

First step: Performance testing and current state analysis

Once the athlete is familiar with the training and racing demands of mountain biking, the next step is to establish his current state of physical fitness. Without this it is very hard to know what kind of training to prescribe. Only once the fitness state is determined can it be assessed whether the envisaged volumes and intensities are at the correct level. A fitness test does not necessarily mean a laboratory-based performance test. A time-trial result, the outcome of your last race or, even simpler, an experienced mountain biker's physical awareness, are enough to give you or other people an idea of your form. If this assessment is incorrect and the training based upon it turns out to be over or under challenging, the plan must be adjusted.

The performance diagnosis should also be accompanied by an analysis of the athlete's general circumstances (i.e., social environment, job).

In addition, previous years of training workload and form development should also be examined as part of the fitness assessment. Excessive annual workload increases in terms of total volume usually have a negative effect on the form development. A race and training analysis of the previous year is the final stage in the evaluation process.

[...]

ISBN: 978-1-78255-014-3

*Available in book stores and on **www.m-m-sports.com***